Rüdiger Martin Zimmerer

Cancer Stem Cell Features In Established Melanoma Cell Lines

Rüdiger Martin Zimmerer

Cancer Stem Cell Features In Established Melanoma Cell Lines

Developing a cancer stem cell model in melanoma cell lines

Südwestdeutscher Verlag für Hochschulschriften

Impressum/Imprint (nur für Deutschland/ only for Germany)
Bibliografische Information der Deutschen Nationalbibliothek: Die Deutsche Nationalbibliothek verzeichnet diese Publikation in der Deutschen Nationalbibliografie; detaillierte bibliografische Daten sind im Internet über http://dnb.d-nb.de abrufbar.

Alle in diesem Buch genannten Marken und Produktnamen unterliegen warenzeichen-, marken- oder patentrechtlichem Schutz bzw. sind Warenzeichen oder eingetragene Warenzeichen der jeweiligen Inhaber. Die Wiedergabe von Marken, Produktnamen, Gebrauchsnamen, Handelsnamen, Warenbezeichnungen u.s.w. in diesem Werk berechtigt auch ohne besondere Kennzeichnung nicht zu der Annahme, dass solche Namen im Sinne der Warenzeichen- und Markenschutzgesetzgebung als frei zu betrachten wären und daher von jedermann benutzt werden dürften.

Verlag: Südwestdeutscher Verlag für Hochschulschriften Aktiengesellschaft & Co. KG
Dudweiler Landstr. 99, 66123 Saarbrücken, Deutschland
Telefon +49 681 37 20 271-1, Telefax +49 681 37 20 271-0
Email: info@svh-verlag.de
Zugl.: Freiburg, Albert-Ludwigs-Universität, Diss., 2009

Herstellung in Deutschland:
Schaltungsdienst Lange o.H.G., Berlin
Books on Demand GmbH, Norderstedt
Reha GmbH, Saarbrücken
Amazon Distribution GmbH, Leipzig
ISBN: 978-3-8381-1367-8

Imprint (only for USA, GB)
Bibliographic information published by the Deutsche Nationalbibliothek: The Deutsche Nationalbibliothek lists this publication in the Deutsche Nationalbibliografie; detailed bibliographic data are available in the Internet at http://dnb.d-nb.de.

Any brand names and product names mentioned in this book are subject to trademark, brand or patent protection and are trademarks or registered trademarks of their respective holders. The use of brand names, product names, common names, trade names, product descriptions etc. even without a particular marking in this works is in no way to be construed to mean that such names may be regarded as unrestricted in respect of trademark and brand protection legislation and could thus be used by anyone.

Publisher: Südwestdeutscher Verlag für Hochschulschriften Aktiengesellschaft & Co. KG
Dudweiler Landstr. 99, 66123 Saarbrücken, Germany
Phone +49 681 37 20 271-1, Fax +49 681 37 20 271-0
Email: info@svh-verlag.de

Printed in the U.S.A.
Printed in the U.K. by (see last page)
ISBN: 978-3-8381-1367-8

Copyright © 2010 by the author and Südwestdeutscher Verlag für Hochschulschriften Aktiengesellschaft & Co. KG and licensors
All rights reserved. Saarbrücken 2010

Aus dem Institut für Chirurgische Forschung und Spitalmanagement des
Universitätsspitals Basel, Schweiz

CANCER STEM CELL FEATURES
IN ESTABLISHED MELANOMA CELL LINES

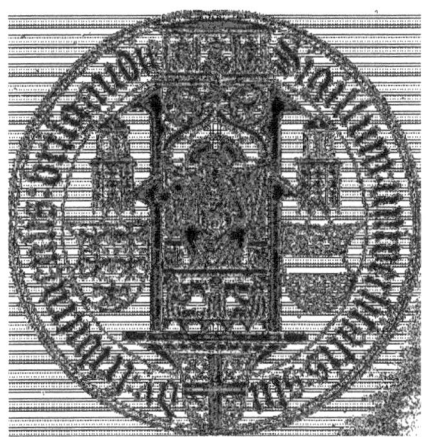

INAUGURAL-DISSERTATION

zur

Erlangung des Medizinischen Doktorgrades
der Medizinischen Fakultät
der Albert-Ludwigs-Universität
Freiburg i. Brg.

2009

Rüdiger Martin Zimmerer

Aalen

Dekan:	Prof. Dr. med. Christoph Peters
1. Gutachter:	Prof. Dr. med. Dr. med. dent. Ralf Schön
2. Gutachter:	Prof. Dr. med. Giulio C Spagnoli
Jahr der Promotion:	2009

TABLE OF CONTENTS

1. ABSTRACT 1
2. TABLE OF FIGURES 3
3. INTRODUCTION 7
   - MALIGNANT MELANOMA 8
   - TREATMENT OF MALIGNANT MELANOMA 9
   - SOMATIC STEM CELLS 10
   - THE CANCER STEM CELL HYPOTHESIS 11
4. AIM OF THE STUDY AND EXPERIMENTAL DESIGN 15
5. MATERIALS AND METHODS 18
   - CULTURE MEDIA AND GROWTH FACTORS 19
   - CULTURE OF MELANOMA CELL LINES 19
   - 3D-CULTURE OF MELANOMA CELL LINES 19
   - GENE EXPRESSION ANALYSIS 20
   - HOX GENE EXPRESSION 24
   - FLUORESCENCE-ACTIVATED CELL SORTING 26
   - IMMUNO-MAGNETIC CELL SEPARATION 26
   - CELL CLONING VIA LIMITED DILUTION ANALYSIS 27
   - GENE EXPRESSION PROFILING 29

6	**RESULTS**	39
	CHARACTERIZATION OF MELANOMA CELL LINES	40
	HOX GENE EXPRESSION	44
	PHENOTYPIC CHARACTERIZATION OF MELANOMA CELL LINES	52
	FUNCTIONAL CHARACTERIZATION OF DIFFERENT CELL LINES	58
	GENE EXPRESSION PROFILING OF CD133+ D10 CELLS	60
	PANTHER CLASSIFICATION SYSTEM	60
7	**DISCUSSION**	77
	SUMMARY	83
8	**SUPPLEMENTARY MATERIAL**	84
	DETAILED PROTOCOL OF TARGET SYNTHESIS	85
9	**REFERENCES**	91
10	**APPENDIX**	107
	ACKNOWLEDGEMENTS	108

ABSTRACT

CANCER STEM CELL FEATURES IN ESTABLISHED MELANOMA CELL LINES

OBJECTIVE
Subpopulations of cancer cells are capable of reproducing tumours in immunocompromised mice. Cancer stem cells (CSC) are usually rare in clinical specimens and hardly amenable to functional studies or to analysis of gene expression profiles. We screened a panel of melanoma cell lines to identify cellular reagents sharing typical CSC features including expression of specific surface markers and genes, capacity to grow in spheroids and high clonogenic capacity.

METHODS:
D10, HBL, Me39, Me59, Me67, MZ2, Na8, RE and WM115 melanoma cell lines were studied. Stem cell associated surface markers were analyzed by flow-cytometry. Clonogenic assays were performed by limiting dilution analysis (LDA) on cells sorted according to expression of selected markers. Gene expression profiles were assessed by using real-time reverse-transcriptase polymerase chain reaction and Affymetrix GeneChip® (Human Genome U133A2.0) arrays.

RESULTS
Na8, D10 and HBL cells, formed spheroids when cultured on plastic coated with poly-HEMA, preventing cell attachment. In all lines except HBL $\geq 75\%$ of cells expressed CD105 but only D10 cell line expressed the classical CSC marker CD133. In contrast, only HBL cell line expressed CD117, a known differentiation marker. In D10 line, CD133+ cells displayed a significantly higher clonogenic capacity as compared to CD133- cells while CD105 expression was not associated with higher clonogenic capacity in any cell line. D10, Me39, RE and WM115 cells expressed at least two of three genes, SOX2, NANOG and OCT4, involved in maintenance of stemness in mesenchymal stem cells. We addressed gene profiling of CD133+ and CD133- D10 cells. We found that 68 genes were up-regulated while 47 genes were down-regulated in CD133+ D10 cells (+/- 1.3 fold, $p < 0.01$), as compared to CD133- cells. Two genes were outstandingly up-regulated, MGP and PROM1 (CD133). A number of other genes up-regulated in CD133+ D10 cells, encode proteins involved in cell proliferation including insulin-like growth factor-1, insulin-like growth factor binding protein 3 and PDGFc. Down-regulated genes included those encoding Tenascin C and TIMP-1.

CONCLUSIONS
Established melanoma cell lines exhibit to variable extents typical features of CSC. D10 cell line, growing in spheroids and expressing CD133 might qualify as a potential "*in vitro*" model of melanoma stem cells.

TABLE OF FIGURES

FIGURE 1 Stem cell hierarchy and analogy of normal stem cells and cancer stem cells. **A** Normal somatic stem cells arise during foetal development. Foetal stem cells self-renew and give rise to form both, daughter stem cells and more differentiated progenies (asymmetric cell division). Adult stem cells either self-renew or undergo multilineage differentiation to maintain the adult tissue. **B** Cancer stem cells might either arise from mutationally transformed normal adult stem cells or from progenitors or differentiated mature cells which acquired cancer stem cell properties such as self-renewal potential. Figure modified from Pardal [Pardal et al. 2003]. 14

FIGURE 2 Experimental design. The panel of melanoma cell lines under investigation includes nine established cell lines. Cells were cultured under different conditions including monolayer expansion in tissue culture flasks and petri dishes; 3D-culture in pre-treated tissue culture flask to prevent cell attachment to the plastic surface. Upon expansion or 3D-culture, melanoma cell lines were investigated for the expression of specific genes and stem cell surface markers. The clonogenic capacity of melanoma cell lines was assessed by limiting dilution analysis (LDA) and Poisson`s Distribution. Gene expression profiling was carried out on sorted CD133+ D10 cells. MAA* = melanoma associated antigens; CTA* = cancer/testis antigens. RegTF** = regulatory core transcription factors NANOG, OCT4, SOX2. 17

FIGURE 3 Clonogenic assays were performed by Limiting dilution analysis (LDA) on cells magnetically sorted according to their expression of selected surface markers Cells were magnetically labelled with MicroBeads® and sorted using a MACS®Separator for magnetic cell separation. Poisson`s Distribution revealed that 41% of CD133+ D10 cells gave rise to clonogenic progenies whereas only 6% of CD133- cells were capable to do so (table). The percentage of negative wells is plotted on the ordinate (y-axis) while the cell concentration is plotted on the abscissa (x-axis). When 37% of the test cultures are negative there is an average of one cell per well, therefore the frequency of proliferating cells with a given phenotype can be extrapolated directly from the graph 28

FIGURE 4 A Results of flow cytometric analysis (FACS) before the actual cell sorting. Histogram (1) and dotplots (2) + (3) of D10 cells, incubated with a monoclonal mouse IgG (Isotype control). Corresponding Histogram and dotplot statistics to graphs of the negative control are displayed in the tables (4) and (5). **B** flow cytometry analysis of CD133 expression in D10. In 4% formaldehyd fixed cells were incubated with anti-CD133 (epitope 2, CD133/2).Histogram (1) and dotplots (2) + (3) of D10 cells, labeled with anti CD133 PE–conjugated monoclonal antibody. More than 90% of gated D10 cells express CD133. Region R2 (69.4%) includes CD133+ cells selected to be sorted by FACS Vantage.Corresponding Histogram and dotplot statistics to the graphs are displayed in the tables (4) and (5). 30

FIGURE 5 A Results of Fluorescent-Activated-Cell-Sorting (FACS) by FACS Vantage. Histogram (1) and dotplots (2) + (3) of sorted CD133+ D10 cells. The fraction of D10 cells positively sorted for CD133 includes more than 97-99% of gated cells (Region R2).Corresponding Histogram and dotplot statistics to the graphs are displayed in the tables (4) and (5). **B** Results of Fluorescent-Activated-Cell-Sorting (FACS) by FACS Vantage. Histogram (1) and dotplots (2) + (3) of sorted CD133- D10 cells. The fraction of CD133- sorted cells includes almost 42% of gated cells (Region R3). Corresponding Histogram and dotplot statistics to the graphs are displayed in the tables (4) and (5). 31

FIGURE 7 Electrophoresis Run Summary. Verification of total RNA isolated from the D10 duplicates, CD133+ [samples (1) + (3)] and CD133- [samples (2) + (4)]. **A** agarose gel, **B** results for ladder (L), **C** standard curve, **D** sample electropherograms use to train RIN. [FU] = fluorescence , [s] = seconds, [nt] = number of nucleotides, RIN = RNA integrity number . The RIN software algorithm (Agilent Technologies) allows for the classification of eukaryotic total RNA, based on a numbering system from 1 to 10, with 10 being the most intact RNA profile. 35

FIGURE 8 Electrophoresis run summary. Verification of cRNA upon fragmentation for target synthesis. Un-fragmented (1, 3, 5, 7) and corresponding fragmented (F) samples (2, 4, 6, 8) of cRNA from CD133+ and CD133- D10 cells, respectively. (L) = ladder, (F) = fragmented cRNA samples, [FU] = fluorescence , [s] = seconds. 37

FIGURE 9 **A** Staining of the probe arrays **B** Affymetrix GeneChip **C** Probe cell distribution. Each gene on the Affymetrix® GeneChip® is represented by a probe set. Each probe set consists of 11-20 probe pairs of oligonucleotides with a length of 25. A probe pair consists of perfect match (PM) and mismatch (MM). Probes that are complementary to the sequence of interest are called perfect match (PM), probes that are complementary to the sequence of interest except for homomeric base change (A-T or G-C) at the 13th position are called mismatch (MM). MM is created by changing the middle (13th) base, to measure non-specific binding. 38

FIGURE 11 Expression of the four HOX loci (HOXA-, -B, -C and –D)in melanoma cells lines. Results of conventional PCR performed on .Each locus is represented by a different colour. The posterior Loci HOXC and HOXD are expressed more frequently in the melanoma cells lines 47

FIGURE 12 HOX gene expression in melanoma cell lines. Results of conventional PCR. Clustered Hox gene organization. The four HOX clusters (HOX A-D) each contain 8–11 genes and are located on four different chromosomes. Each gene is represented by a coloured box. Individual genes in different HOX clusters can be aligned into paralogous groups (identical colours) based on the sequence homology within their homeobox regions. Beyond each HOX cluster the corresponding status of HOX gene expression in melanoma cell lines; red = active gene; blue = inactive gene. 49

FIGURE 13 Quantitative Real-Time RT-PCR of HOX Expression in Melanoma cell lines. **A** HOXA13; **B** HOXB7; **C** HOXB13; **D** HOXC8; **E** HOXC9; **F** HOXC10. Calibrator sample represents the unitary amount of the target of interest, the other samples express n-fold mRNA relative to the calibrator. Final amounts of target were determined as follows: target amount = 2^{-Ct}, where Ct = [Ct (HOXgene) – Ct (ACTB)]sample – [Ct (HOXgene) – Ct (ACTB)]calibrator. 50

FIGURE 14 Quantitative Real-Time RT-PCR of HOX Expression in Melanoma cell lines. **G** HOXC11; **H** HOXC12; **I** HOXC13; **K** HOXD9; **L** HOXD13. Calibrator sample represents the unitary amount of the target of interest, the other samples express n-fold mRNA relative to the calibrator. Final amounts of target were determined as follows: target amount = 2^{-Ct}, where Ct = [Ct (HOXgene) – Ct (ACTB)]sample – [Ct (HOXgene) – Ct (ACTB)]calibrator. 51

FIGURE 15 Phenotype of D10 cell line. Expression levels of APC-conjugated monoclonal antibodies against the CD133 epitope (red graph). 55

FIGURE 16 Na8 spheroids in polyHEMA-coated tissue culture flask. A = 2x magnification, B = 4x magnifictaion, C = 40x magnification..57

FIGURE 17 Results of PANTHER analysis performed on 65 up-regulated genes in CD133+ D10 cells. Molecular function A and biological process B those 65 genes are involved in. 63

FIGURE 18 Results of PANTHER analysis performed on 44 down-regulated genes in CD133+ D10 65

INTRODUCTION

MALIGNANT MELANOMA

Melanoma of the skin captures 5% in men and 4% in women of estimated cancer cases in the USA for 2008. The age-adjusted incidence of malignant melanoma is region-dependent and quotes 40 in Australia, 19 in the United States, 14 in central Europe and 1-3 in Asia and the Orient per 100.000 individuals per anum. There has been a 50% increase in the melanoma incidence since 1975. According to the WHO World Cancer Report, 48.000 melanoma related deaths occur worldwide per annum. Malignant melanoma is caused by mutationally transformed melanocytes which are found predominantly in skin but also in the bowel and the eye (uveal melanoma). The main aetiologies promoting skin melanoma development can be assigned to three groups: firstly, dispositional factors, including race (caucasian ethnicity), type of skin (skin type I/II), albinism and a positive family history of melanoma, secondly, acquired factors involving sunburn history and multifactorial immune deficiencies and, finally, precursor lesions including atypical naevi and congenital naevi. There is a 64-fold higher risk of developing melanoma with more than 50 naevi. Epidemiological data suggest that exposure to ultraviolet radiation [Situm et al. 2007] (UVA and UVB) is one of the major contributors to the development of melanoma, mostly due more to intermittent extreme UV exposure and associated sunburns than to continuous and constant UV radiation. Melanoma is most common on the back in men and on legs in women (areas of occasional sun exposure). The individual risk for developing melanoma appears to be strongly influenced by socio-economic conditions rather than indoor versus outdoor occupations. It is more common in professional and administrative workers than unskilled workers. Basically, there are four different types of malignant melanoma of the skin, differing in clinical and histopathological features (**TABLE 1**). The most common type is the superficially spreading melanoma (SSM) capturing almost 58% of all cutaneous melanomas. SSM initially infiltrates the skin/epidermis horizontally and subsequently progresses and distributes in vertical direction subcutaneously. In contrast, the nodular malignant melanoma (NMM), the fastest growing entity, predominately invades tissues vertically. The lentigo maligna melanoma (LMM) occurs in light-exposed areas and it is associated which a higher median incidence age and distinguished by slow growth. Palmar and plantar melanomas rank among the acral lentiginous melanoma (ALM) and are the most common type of melanoma in Africa and Asia. Histologically, they either can be SSM or NMM.

TABLE 1	SUBTYPES OF PRIMARY MALIGNANT MELANOMA	
Subtype	Percentage (%)	Median age (years)
SSM	57,4	51
NMM	21,4	56
LMM	8,8	68
ALM	4,0	63

Clinical and histological subtypes of primary malignant melanoma in German speaking countries. **SSM** = superficial spreading melanoma; **NMM** = nodular malignant melanoma; **LMM** = lentigo malignant melanoma, **ALM** = acral lentiginous melanoma.

TREATMENT OF MALIGNANT MELANOMA

According to the evidence and interdisciplinary consensus-based German guidelines, the primary treatment of a melanoma is surgical excision. An excisional biopsy is preferred, and safety margins of 1 cm for tumour thickness up to 2 mm and 2 cm for higher tumour thickness should be applied either at primary excision or in a two-step procedure. The sentinel lymph node biopsy should be performed in patients whose primary melanoma is thicker than 1.0 mm. In clinically identified lymph node metastases, radical lymph node dissection is considered standard therapy. If distant metastases involve just one internal organ and operative removal is feasible, then surgery should be seen as therapy of choice. Radiation therapy for the primary treatment of melanoma is indicated only in those cases in which surgery is impossible or not reasonable. In regional lymph nodes, radiation therapy is usually recommended when excision is not complete (R1 resection) or if the nodes are inoperable. In distant metastases, radiation therapy is particularly indicated in bone metastases, brain metastases and soft tissue metastases. Systemic medical treatment of melanoma is administered in the adjuvant and palliative setting. Adjuvant therapy may be considered in patients with primary melanoma with more than 1.5 mm tumour thickness and with regional node metastasis. Presently, no consensus for systemic adjuvant chemotherapy or for adjuvant therapy with nonspecific immune-stimulatory agents outside controlled studies has been reached. Interferon-alpha is the first substance in the adjuvant therapy of melanoma, which has shown a significant clinical benefit to the patients in some prospective randomized studies. Good arguments for using adjuvant interferon-alpha therapy in high-risk melanoma patients exist. Both, high-dose and low-dose interferon-alpha therapy show promise. The major indications for systemic chemotherapy and chemoimmunotherapy are inoperable recurrent tumours, inoperable regional metastases and distant metastases (stage IV). As treatment in such situations is primarily palliative, the effect of any regimen on the quality of life must be carefully weighed. As a first line treatment, single agent therapy is recommended, as polychemotherapy or biochemotherapy did not show significant advantages for prolongation of survival and they are associated with higher toxicity [Garbe et al. 2008b, Garbe et al. 2008a, Garbe et al. 2008c]. Patients with advanced disease have a poor prognosis with a reported median survival ranging between 3 and 11 months [Rietschel et al. 2008].

SOMATIC STEM CELLS

Somatic stem cells are self-renewing, typically multipotent, progenitors with the broadest developmental potential in a particular tissue, at a particular time. Self-renewal is the process by which a progenitor cell gives rise to daughter progenitors of equivalent developmental potential. For example, multipotent stem cells self-renew by dividing to generate one or two multipotent daughter cells. Progenitors include both, stem cells and restricted progenitors. A restricted progenitor is a cell that divides to give rise to other cells, but which has a more limited developmental potential. Somatic stem cells arise from embryonic precursors during foetal development. Embryonic stem cells (ES) or foetal stem cells (FS) from the inner cell mass of early embryo are considered to be pluripotent cells and are thus able to differentiate towards all different specific cell types of an adult organism. Foetal stem cells themselves self-renew to form daughter cells and differentiate to generate diverse mature progeny including adult stem cells, which often continue to self-renew and undergo multilineage differentiation to maintain the adult tissues they originally derive from. Dellatore and colleagues [Dellatore et al. 2008] have emphasized the importance of the niche in terms of regulating lineage-specific stem cell self-renewal. Niches are composed of supportive cells and the extracellular matrix components which are arranged in a 3D topography of controlled stiffness in the presence of oxygen and growth factor gradients.

THE CANCER STEM CELL HYPOTHESIS

Parallels have been drawn between somatic stem cells and cancer cells. They share many common features, in particular, both types of cells may be able to self-renew and differentiate. However, contrary to somatic stem cells, cancer cells self-renew and differentiate in an uncontrolled and abnormal manner. In teratocarcinoma, medulloblastoma and myeloid leukaemia both differentiated and undifferentiated tumour cells coexist. For instance, teratocarcinoma may give rise to highly differentiated tissue types including bone, cartilage, teeth and hair besides undifferentiated cancer cells [Sell 1993; Sell 2004; Sell, Pierce 1994]. Subsets of medulloblastoma cells were reported to resemble neurons and glia [Wechsler-Reya 2001; Wechsler-Reya, Scott 2001] and myeloid leukaemia cells were shown to differentiate towards several lineages of blood cells [Fearon et al. 1986b, Fearon et al. 1986a].

Assays focusing on the ability of tumour cells to transplant cancers in immunodeficient hosts have shown that only a small subpopulation of malignant cells is able to do so [Reya et al. 2001]. The idea that tumours comprise cells endowed with heterogeneous tumourigenicity and differentiation potential [Hamburger, Salmon 1977] is reflected by the biology of teratocarcinoma. However, still unclear is whether this idea can also apply to more common malignancies. By applying the principles of stem cell biology to cancer many tumours have recently been shown to be organized hierarchically into clonally derived populations of cells with different tumourigenic potentials (**FIGURE 1**). For example, Bonnet and colleagues [Bonnet, Dick 1997] were the first who could phenotypically distinguish cells of AML (acute myeloid leukaemia) with high tumourigenicity from the remaining tumour cells using surface markers. Following the proof of existence of CSC in AML, similar reports were made for breast cancer [Al-Hajj et al. 2003] and medulloblastoma [Singh et al. 2003]. Both studies demonstrated that not all human breast and brain cancer cells were equal in terms of their ability to form colonies in culture and to reproduce tumours *in vivo* and that there are subsets of tumour cells exhibiting properties of cancer stem cells. In particular, a high self-renewal potential, coupled with the capacity to differentiate and generate phenotypically diverse cancer cells was observed. Mutations that deregulate pathways controlling normal stem cell self-renewal, such as the WNT, sonic hedgehog (SHH), Notch, PTEN and BMI1 pathways, also regulate proliferation of cancer stem cells causing diverse range of cancers [Reya et al.

2001; Taipale, Beachy 2001; Zhu, Parada 2002]. For example, malignant transformation in the WNT signalling pathway, promoting self-renewal of haematopoietic stem cells [Willert et al. 2003; Austin et al. 1997; Murdoch et al. 2003] may lead, depending on the mutated stem cell involved, to lymphoblastic leukaemia [Chung et al. 2002; Qiang et al. 2003], colorectal cancer [van de Wetering et al. 2002], pilomatricoma [Gat et al. 1998; Chan et al. 1999] and medulloblastoma [Zurawel et al. 1998]. This suggests that cancer can be considered a disease of unregulated self-renewal and tumours may arise from the self-renewal and differentiation of cancer stem cells possibly following mutations affecting self-renewal pathways of somatic stem cells (**FIGURE 1**). The observation that tumours often relapse or metastasize upon chemotherapy despite complete regression of the primary tumour might be explained by the fact that cancer stem cells are more likely to express drug resistance and anti-apoptotic proteins and are more resistant to chemotherapies than differentiated cancer cells. As previously mentioned, the existence of CSC was first clearly documented in the context of leukaemia where only a minor percentage of leukaemic cells were able to proliferate extensively *in vitro* and *in vivo*. The question whether every leukaemic cell had the same proliferation rate or whether there were differences among the leukaemic cells from the same patient in terms of the ability to proliferate was first answered by Dick's group [Bonnet, Dick 1997] who showed that only a small subset of AML, phenotypically similar to haematopoietic stem cells, could transfer AML when transplanted into immunodeficient mice. Other AML cells failed to reconstitute the tumour and to induce leukaemia upon transplantation. This was extended by Al-Hajj and colleagues [Al-Hajj et al. 2003] who could show that not all human breast cancer cells had the ability to form tumours in immunocompromised mice. It was suggested that the tumourigenic cell population represented a minority of cells within the tumour, and that its isolation could be attempted from most tumours based on a unique surface marker expression pattern. A few properties of cancer stem cells have been identified so far, including their common capacity to grow in anti-adhesive structures called spheroids and a higher resistance to hypoxia, possibly related to aberrant angiogenesis in rapidly expanding tumours [Carmeliet, Jain 2000; Pouysségur et al. 2006]. Fang [Fang et al. 2005] described a subset of cells derived from freshly isolated or in vitro stabilized melanoma cell lines that was able to form "melanoma spheroids" when grown in a specific stem cell medium. Tavaluc [Tavaluc et al. 2007] and Zhou [Zhou, Zhang 2008] suggest that cancer stem cells have a higher ability to survive under hypoxic conditions than normal cancer cells. Current cancer therapeutics based on tumour regression may target and kill differentiated tumour cells, which compose the bulk of the tumour, while sparing the rare cancer stem cell population. The cancer stem cell model suggests that the design of new cancer therapeutics may require the targeting and elimination of cancer stem cells. Therefore, it is imperative to design new strategies based upon a better understanding of the signalling pathways that control aspects of self-renewal and survival in cancer stem cells in order to identify novel therapeutic targets in these cell.

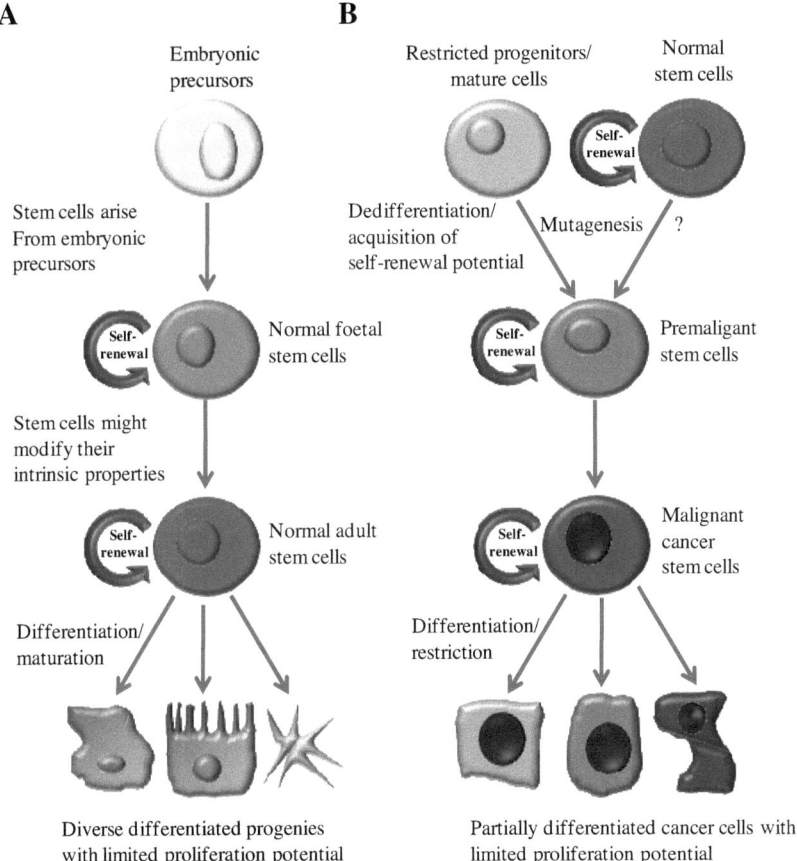

FIGURE 1 Stem cell hierarchy and analogy of normal stem cells and cancer stem cells. **A** Normal somatic stem cells arise during foetal development. Foetal stem cells self-renew and give rise to form both, daughter stem cells and more differentiated progenies (asymmetric cell division). Adult stem cells either self-renew or undergo multilineage differentiation to maintain the adult tissue. **B** Cancer stem cells might either arise from mutationally transformed normal adult stem cells or from progenitors or differentiated mature cells which acquired cancer stem cell properties such as self-renewal potential. Figure modified from Pardal [Pardal et al. 2003].

AIM OF THE STUDY AND EXPERIMENTAL DESIGN

AIM OF THE STUDY

Cancer stem cells (CSC) markers, potentially allowing the functional characterization of specific cell subsets from clinical specimens, have been identified in different types of tumours, including melanoma [Schatton et al. 2008].

However, the minute numbers of cells presenting these features that can be obtained from surgical samples usually prevent a thorough evaluation of the molecular pathways involved in "stemness". This background has prompted several research groups to explore the possibility of taking advantage of the relative heterogeneity of established cells lines to identify cell subsets endowed with CSC features.

In this work we have addressed typical CSC phenotypical and functional features in melanoma cell lines, in order to identify cellular reagents amenable to detailed molecular profiling. The experimental strategy adopted in this study is outlined in **FIGURE 2** on the following page.

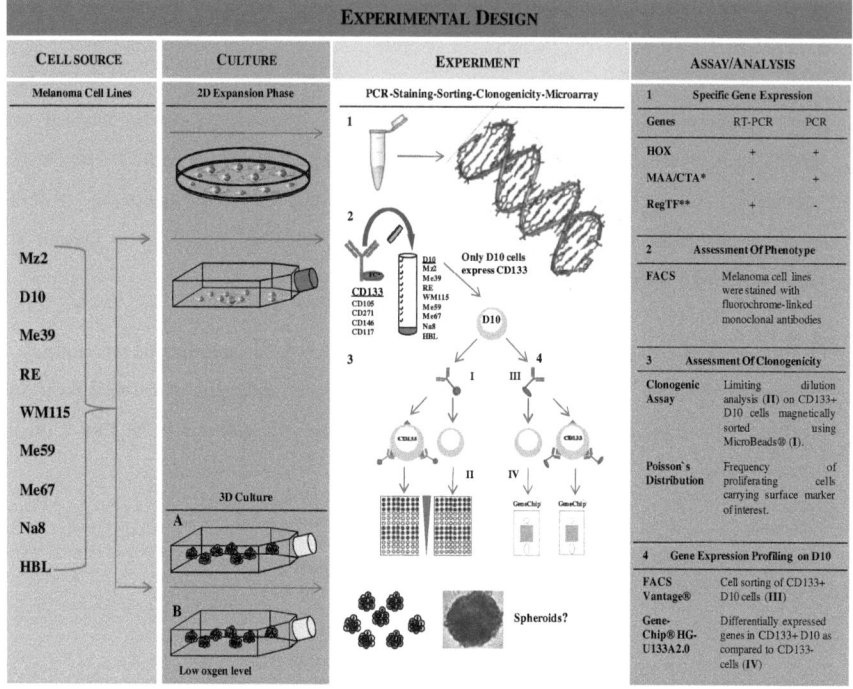

FIGURE 2 Experimental design. The panel of melanoma cell lines under investigation includes nine established cell lines. Cells were cultured under different conditions including monolayer expansion in tissue culture flasks and petri dishes; 3D-culture in pre-treated tissue culture flask to prevent cell attachment to the plastic surface. Upon expansion or 3D-culture, melanoma cell lines were investigated for the expression of specific genes and stem cell surface markers. The clonogenic capacity of melanoma cell lines was assessed by limiting dilution analysis (LDA) and Poisson`s Distribution. Gene expression profiling was carried out on sorted CD133+ D10 cells. **MAA*** = melanoma associated antigens; **CTA*** = cancer/testis antigens. **RegTF**** = regulatory core transcription factors NANOG, OCT4, SOX2.

MATERIALS AND METHODS

CULTURE MEDIA AND GROWTH FACTORS

Melanoma cell lines under investigation were cultured and expanded in GIBCO`s DMEM (Invitrogen AG, Basel, Switzerland, containing 4.5g/L Glucose and NEAA), supplemented with 10% fetal bovine serum (FBS, Invitrogen AG, Basel, Switzerland), 1% sodium pyruvate (Invitrogen AG, Basel, Switzerland), 1% HEPES buffer (Invitrogen AG, Basel, Switzerland) and 2% PSG (penicillin, streptomycin, gentamycin, Invitrogen AG, Basel, Switzerland), thereafter referred to as complete DMEM (cDMEM) in this work.

CULTURE OF MELANOMA CELL LINES

A selection of nine human melanoma cell lines, originally derived from metastatic melanomas, stored frozen in liquid nitrogen, were thawed in 37°C water bath and immediately resuspended in cDMEM. After 10min recovery phase, cells were centrifuged at 1400rpm for 4min, resuspended in cDMEM and plated in 150cm^2 tissue cultured flasks. When cells reached confluence, they were detached with 0.05% trypsin with 0.01 EDTA (Invitrogen AG, Basel, Switzerland) counted and plated in again. The melanoma cell lines MZ2, Me39 and D10 were seeded at 500 cells/cm^2, WM115 and RE at 700 cells/cm2, Me59 and Me67 at 1000 cells/cm^2. When necessary cells were frozen.

3D-CULTURE OF MELANOMA CELL LINES

CULTURE IN POLYHEMA-COATED FLASKS

Some cancer stem cells have been reported to grow in 3D-structures when attachment to plastic culture flasks is prevented. Na8 and HBL cells were published by our group to generate such spheroids and as an empiric approach, all melanoma cell lines under investigation were cultured 75cm^2 tissue culture flasks (TPP, MIDSCI, St. Louis, MO, USA) treated with PolyHEMA (Poly2-hydroxyethylmethacrylate, Sigma-Aldrich®, St. Louis, MO, USA) preventing the attachment of cells to the plastic. Due to the fact that low oxygen level atmosphere was reported to promote stem cell growth, melanoma cell lines were also cultured in both, 20% and 1% oxygen humidified atmosphere at 37°C in PolyHEMA-coated tissue culture flasks.

PolyHEMA granules were dissolved in 100% ethanol at 120mg/ml in an evaporation preventing glass bottle overnight at 37°C on an orbital shaker. The homogenous solution was diluted to a final concentration of 50mg/ml with 100% ethanol the following day and incubated again at 37°C on an orbital shaker for two hours. Tissue culture flasks were coated with 5ml PolyHEMA solution under laminar flow bench and they were left open to allow ethanol evaporation and polymerization of PolyHEMA solution on the bottom of the tissue culture flasks. The next day all melanoma cell lines were seeded at 5×10^4 cells/ml in cDMEM and each cell line was incubated in 20% and 1% oxygen atmosphere at 37°C.

GENE EXPRESSION ANALYSIS

Melanoma cell lines were investigated for the expression of the genes encoding the regulatory core transcription factors NANOG, OCT4 and SOX2, The expression of these genes was assessed by using quantitative Real-Time RT-PCR. The expression of the genes encoding the melanoma associated antigens (MAA) gp100, tyrosinase and Melan-A/MART-1 and the cancer/testis antigens (CTA) MAGE-3 and NY-ESO was assessed by conventional PCR and its extent was semiquantitatively evaluated by densitometry [Spagnoli et al. 1995]. Primers and probes for the housekeeping gene ß-actin (hACTB) as well as for NANOG, OCT4, SOX2 and MAGE-3 were provided by Assays-on-Demand, Gene Expression Products (Applied Biosystems, Foster City, CA, USA). The other primer sequences (gp100, tyrosinase, Melan-A/MART-1 and NY-ESO) were derived from existing literature, as indicated below or were generated using appropriate software (Primer Express™, Applied Biosystems, Foster City, CA). Sequences of primers and probes are reported in **TABLE 2**, Assays on-Demand in **TABLE 3**. The analysis of the HOX gene expression in melanoma cell lines is described separately in this chapter.

RNA EXTRACTION

RNA extraction procedures were carried out on ice in RNAse free environment. Thawed samples were sonicated for 60s, diluted with Trizol (Invitrogen AG, Basel, Switzerland) and then incubated on ice for 10min. Following centrifugation at 11.000rpm for 15min two phases resulted. The upper aqueous phase was transferred to a fresh microfuge tubes containing 2μl glycogen ($20\mu g/\mu$l, Invitrogen AG, Basel, Switzerland). To allow RNA precipitation, 125μl isopropanol (100%, Hänseler AG, Herisau, Switzerland) were added to the solution, the tubes were vortexed, incubated on ice for 5-10 minutes and finally spun again at 11.000rpm for 10min. The isopropanol supernatant was discarded by inversion and the tubes were blotted dry on a sterile paper. Finally, the resulting pellets were washed at least three times with 250μl ethanol (75%, Pharmacy, University Hospital, Basel, Switzerland) whereas the pellets were detached by vortexing and the tubes were centrifuged at 11.000rpm for 5min. After the third washing procedure residual ethanol was removed by air drying. Pellets were dissolved in 35μl DEPC–treated H_2O (100μl of 0.1% Diethylpyrocarbonate (Sigma-Aldrich, Steinheim, Germany) to 100ml milliQ H_2O)) in a heating block set at 60°C for 1min and immediately put on ice.

RNA MEASUREMENT

The RNA concentration of each sample was measured with a spectrophotometer at a wavelength of 260nm. According to the spectrophotometer analysis RNA concentration of each sample was calculated and a purity index was determined as fraction of the optical density (OD) at 260nm and 280nm. Acceptable ranges were considered to be >1.5.

TREATMENT WITH DNASE

Since genomic DNA contamination can lead to false positive real-time RT-PCR results DNase treatment on the RNA samples was performed. Briefly, following RNA measurement 5μg RNA and DNase Mix (1μl DNase and 2μl (10x) DNase buffer, both Ambion Inc., Austin, TX, USA) were added to a RNase free microfuge tube and placed for 30 minutes at 37°C in a water bath. Following the incubation in the water bath, samples were immediately put back on ice. The DNase was inactivated using a concentrated DNase Inactivator (Ambion Inc., Austin, TX, USA). The reaction took place at room temperature for 2min. The samples were mixed by vortexing and centrifuged for 1min at 1600rpm.

REVERSE TRANSCRIPTION

DNase-free RNA was reverse transcribed into cDNA. A series of RNase-free tubes was preloaded with 1μl Random Primer (Promega Corp., Madison, WI, USA) and 19μl RNA was added to the samples. Samples were incubated at 70°C for 10min in a heating block.

Meanwhile, the master mix for cDNA transcription was prepared, comprising 1μl Stratascript Reverse Transcriptase Enzyme (Invitrogen AG, Basel, Switzerland), 2.0μl of a 10mM desoxyribonukleosidtriphosphate mix (dNTP, including 2.5mM of each of the four bases: dATP, dCTP, dGTP and dTTP, Invitrogen AG, Basel, Switzerland), 2.8μl of 10x concentrated buffer (Invitrogen AG, Basel, Switzerland) and 2.2μl DEPC-treated H$_2$O. The tubes were placed in a thermal cycler for polymerization (15min at 25°C → 30min at 42°C → 20min at 48°C → 15min at 70°C). After polymerization, RNA stock was diluted 1:20 for Quantitative Real-Time Reverse-Transcriptase Polymerase Chain reaction (qReal-Time RT-PCR). The quality of obtained cDNA was assessed by checking the expression of the house keeping gene ß-actin (hACTB) according to established protocols.

QUANTITATIVE REAL-TIME RT-PCR

PCR reactions were performed and monitored by using the ABI Prism 7700 Sequence Detection System (Perkin Elmer/Applied Biosystems, Rotkreuz, Switzerland). The PCR master mix was based on AmpliTaq Gold DNA polymerase (Perkin Elmer/Applied Biosystems). In the same reaction, cDNA samples (5 μl, for a total volume of 25 μl per reaction) were analyzed both for the gene of interest and for the reference gene (18S ribosomal RNA [rRNA] or hACTB), using a multiplex approach (Perkin Elmer/Applied Biosystems User Bulletin no. 2). The probe for hACTB was fluorescently labelled with VIC (Perkin Elmer/Applied Biosystems) and 6-carboxytetramethylrhodamine (TAMRA); probes for genes of interest were labelled with 6-carboxyfluorescein and TAMRA. Primers and probes used for gp100, tyrosinase, Melan/Mart-1 and NY-ESO are reported in **TABLE 2**. Assays-on-Demand were available for the primers and probes used for hACTB, NANOG, OCT4 and SOX2 (**TABLE 3**).The total reaction volume of 25μl was loaded in duplicate wells from 96-well-plates, which were centrifuged at 1500rpm for 1 min. The PCR was run with cycle temperatures and times described by Martin and his group [Martin et al. 2001]. The Ct value of a real-time PCR reaction corresponds to the cycle number where the fluorescence intensity reaches a threshold (usually, in the range 0.03-0.06). The threshold level was selected to include all amplification curves in their exponential phase. For each cDNA sample, the threshold cycle (Ct) value of each target sequence was subtracted from the Ct value of the reference gene to derive ΔCt. The level of expression of each target gene was then calculated as 2ΔCt. Each sample was tested at least twice for each gene of interest.

TABLE 2   DESCRIPTION OF THE DESIGNED PRIMERS & PROBES FOR REAL-TIME RT-PCR*

Gene	Forward and reverse primers (5`→3`)	Probe (5`→3`)
18S rRNA	CGGCTACCACATCCAAGAA GCTGGAATTACCGCGGCT	TGCTGGCACCAGACTTGCCCTC
gp100	TCCCCCTGGATTGTCTTCTG CTCAAATGCATCCCCCTCA	CCCTGGACATTGTCCAGGGTATTGAAAGTGA
MART-1	TCTATGGTTACCCCAAGAAGGG GATCACTGTCAGGATGCCGA	ACGGCTGAAGAGGCCGCTGGGAT
tyrosinase	TTTGCCTGAGTTTGACCCAAT AGAGGCATCCGCTATCCCA	TAGAAATACACTGGAAGGATTTGCTAGTCCACTTACTA
NY-ESO	GCTGAATGGATGCTGCAGA CTGGAGACAGGAGCTGATGGA	TGTGTCCGGCAACATACTGACTATCCGA

*RT-PCR = reverse transcriptase polymerase chain reaction; **rRNA** = ribosomal RNA; **gp100** = melanosomal matrix protein gp100; **MART-1** = Melan/MART-1 = melanoma antigen recognized by T cells; **tyrosinase** = key enzyme in melanin biosynthesis; **NY-ESO** = cancer/testis antigen (see text).

Hox Gene Expression

RNA EXTRACTION AND CDNA SYNTHESIS

Regarding the expression of Homeobox genes (Hox genes), total RNA was isolated from all melanoma cell lines using RNeasy Mini Kit (Qiagen GmbH, Hilden, Germany) following the manufacturer 's instructions and all samples were treated with RNase-free DNase (Qiagen GmbH, Hilden, Germany) to prevent amplification of genomic DNA, as detailed above. The concentration of RNA and the ratio of absorbance at 260nm to 280 nm were measured by the average of triplicate reading using NanoDrop® ND-1000 spectrophotometer (NanoDrop® Technologies, Montchanin, DE, USA). 1 µg RNA was reverse transcribed using Ready-To-Go You-Prime First-Strand Beads (GE Healthcare, Buckinghamshire, UK), according to the manufacturer's protocol using random hexamers (GeneAmp RNA PCR Random Hexamers Set N808-0127 Applied Biosystems, Foster City, CA, USA) as primers.

PCR AMPLIFICATION

PCR amplification of cDNA was performed in a reaction mixture (Pure Taq Ready to go PCR-beads Amersham Biosciences cod. 27-9558-01) containing 4μl of cDNA sample and different primer sets (20p/mol each). The sense/anti-sense HOX primers for PCR were designed as previously reported [Cantile et al. 2003]. To prevent genomic DNA contamination, sense and anti-sense primers were designed to frame a sequence that crossed at least one intron on the genes. The co-amplification of each specific gene and hACTB gene, as an internal control, was achieved using two primer sets in a single reaction mixture. We selected two pairs of hACTB primers to obtain amplified fragments with different molecular weight (149 and 433bp), to be used alternatively in the co-amplification reaction. Duplex-PCR products were separated by ethidium 1.2% agarose gel electrophoresis.

QUANTITATIVE REAL-TIME RT-PCR

TaqMan® analysis was carried out on a 7900HT Sequence Detection System. Singleplex PCR reactions were performed in Fast Gene Quantification in 96-Well Plates (the thermal cycling conditions included a step of 20s at 95°C followed by 40 cycles of 95°C for 1s and 60°C for 20s) with The TaqMan® Fast Universal PCR Master Mix (10 µl) in a volume of 20 µl containing 2µl of cDNA and 1µl of specific TaqMan® Gene Expression Assays for HOX genes (**TABLE 3**), according to the manufacturer's directions. All reactions were performed in triplicate. All reagents were from Applied Biosystems (Foster City, CA, USA). The comparative Ct method [Pfaffl 2001] was employed to determine the differential expression of HOX genes in the cell lines under investigation, using as reference gene hACTB control (Applied Biosystems, Foster City, CA, USA). A calibrator sample was identified that represents the unitary amount of the target of interest; the other samples express n-fold mRNA relative to the calibrator. Final amounts of target were determined as follows: target amount = 2^{-Ct}, where $C_t = [C_t (HOXgene) - C_t (ACTB)]_{sample} - [C_t (HOXgene) - C_t (ACTB)]_{calibrator}$.

TABLE 3 GENE EXPRESSION ASSAYS* FOR REAL-TIME RT-PCR**

HOX genes	AB Assay ID	Gene Symbols	AB Assay ID
HOXA13	Hs00426284_m1	hACTB	Hs99999903_m1
HOXB7	Hs00270131_m1		
HOXB13	Hs00197189_m1	NANOG	Hs02387400_g1
HOXC8	Hs00224073_m1		
HOXC9	Hs00396786_m1	OCT4	Hs00742896_s1
HOXC10	Hs00213579_m1		
HOXC11	Hs00204415_m1	SOX2	Hs00602736_s1
HOXC12	Hs00545229_m1		
HOXC13	Hs00600868_m1	MAGE3	Hs00366532_m1
HOXD9	Hs00610725_m1		
HOXD13	Hs00171253_m1		

*TaqMan® Gene Expression Assays (Assay-on-demand®; see Assay IDs), Applied Biosystems (AB), Foster City, CA.**RT-PCR = reverse-transcriptase polymerase chain reaction; **hACTB** = human ACTB (beta actin) endogenous control; **NANOG** = nanog homeobox; **OCT4** = POU-domain transcription factor; **SOX2** = SRY (sex determining region Y)-box 2; **MAGE3** = melanoma antigen-A3 family.

FLUORESCENCE-ACTIVATED CELL SORTING

Melanoma cell lines were evaluated for their expression of surface markers known to be expressed on stem cells, progenitor cells and cells showing stem cell like behaviour. Cell suspensions from melanoma cell lines were incubated with the following fluorochrome conjugated antibodies: PE/APC-CD133, FITC-CD105, APC-CD271, FITC-CD146 and APC-CD117 (Becton-Dickinson, San José, CA, USA) in 5ml polyethylene tubes in 200µl cDMEM. Between 5×10^5 and 10^6 cells per tube were labelled with 5μl of labelled monoclonal antibodies of interest. Following 45min of antibody incubation protected from light at 4°C, tubes were filled up with 1ml PBS, vortexed and centrifuged at 1400rpm for 4min. The washing procedure was repeated twice. Finally, cells were fixed by resuspension in 500µl of 1% paraformaldehyd (PAF) and the samples were stored at 4°C in the dark until analysis. The phenotype of melanoma cell lines was assessed by flow cytometry using a FACSCalibur® flow cytometer (Becton-Dickinson). Results are expressed as percentages of cells within a gated cell population positive for the surface marker of interest. In order to estimate the density of the expression of surface marker of interest, the mean fluorescence intensity (MFI) was also measured.

IMMUNO-MAGNETIC CELL SEPARATION

In order to assess possible differences in the clonogenic capacity of cells carrying selected surface markers, melanoma cell lines were incubated with MicroBeads® loaded with CD105, CD133, CD271 and CD117 specific monoclonal antibodies (Miltenyi Biotec, http://www.miltenyi.com) and then applied to columns allowing their magnetic separation into positively and negatively labelled fractions by using a MiniMACS™ separation unit (Miltenyi Biotec, http://www.miltenyi.com) according to established protocols. After separation cells were resuspended in 1ml MACS buffer (PBS/0.5% FBS/ 2.5 µM EDTA) and counted with a nuclear stain.

CELL CLONING VIA LIMITED DILUTION ANALYSIS

INTRODUCTION

Limiting dilution assays (LDA) are designed to define the frequency of cells endowed with specific features within a heterogeneous population, e.g., in this study, the frequency of proliferating cells carrying a surface marker of interest. Multiple cultures are set up at different cell concentrations. The fraction of negative cultures is plotted on the ordinate while the cell concentration is plotted on the abscissa to give a straight line. Suitable statistical tests are used to fit this line, including regression analysis and the least square method [Sharrock et al. 1990; Taswell 1981; Svedmyr et al. 1984; Frisan et al. 2001].

LIMITING DILUTION ANALYSIS

Cloning cells by limiting dilution is a procedure for separating cells based on the assumption that if a suspension of cells is diluted with enough culture medium a concentration of cells will be produced such that an accurately measured volume of the diluted suspension will contain 1 single cell. When this volume of the diluted cell suspension is placed into separate wells of a 96-well-plate, each well should receive 1 cell per well. Because each cell type divides differently and this might lead to different cloning efficiencies, cells were distributed over the 96– well-plate at decreasing concentrations. In this study, cell suspensions of melanoma cell lines were diluted serially in 4 increments, whereby cells of each increment were plated in 24 wells (3 rows) of a 96-well-plate. Melanoma cell lines were cultured in cDMEM and the medium was changed dependent on the proliferation rate. Cell counts were carried out twice a week and the experiment was terminated when the cell counts remained unmodified. **FIGURE 3** reports the design of these experiments.

POISSON`S DISTRIBUTION

Poisson`s distribution addresses the probability of a number of results occurring in a fixed period of time in a random experiment. There are only two possible results: success (positive) or not (negative). If the probability of "success" is expected to be little and if the random experiment is repeated quite frequent, Poisson`s Distribution is an approximation to the real probability of the positive result (success). In this study positive results were determined as at least one cell colony with more than 50 cells in one well of each concentration-unit (positive wells). Three rows (24 wells) of a 96-well-plate usually represented a certain cell concentration. Positive results of each 24-well-unit were counted, transformed into percentage of negative wells. The evaluation of the frequency of proliferating cells for each target phenotype was performed by plotting the logarithm of the percentage of negative wells on the Y axis and the cell dilution on the X axis. The zero term of the Poisson equation predicts that when 37% of the test cultures are negative this corresponds to an average of one cell per well, therefore the frequency of proliferating cells with a given phenotype can be extrapolated directly from the graph as shown in a typical result in **FIGURE 3**.

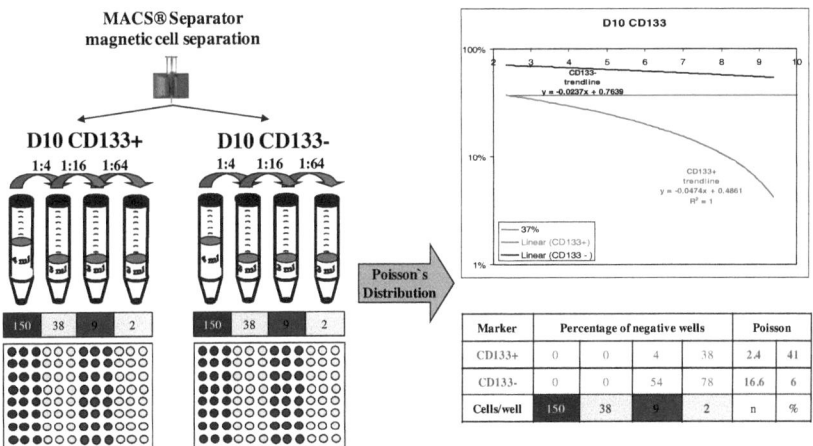

FIGURE 3 Clonogenic assays were performed by Limiting dilution analysis (LDA) on cells magnetically sorted according to their expression of selected surface markers Cells were magnetically labelled with MicroBeads® and sorted using a MACS®Separator for magnetic cell separation. Poisson`s Distribution revealed that 41% of CD133+ D10 cells gave rise to clonogenic progenies whereas only 6% of CD133- cells were capable to do so (table). The percentage of negative wells is plotted on the ordinate (y-axis) while the cell concentration is plotted on the abscissa (x-axis). When 37% of the test cultures are negative there is an average of one cell per well, therefore the frequency of proliferating cells with a given phenotype can be extrapolated directly from the graph

GENE EXPRESSION PROFILING

FACSVANTAGE® CELL SORTING

In order to reveal differences in gene expression of CD133+ and CD133- D10 cells, which might help to understand the function of CD133 as a potential cancer stem cell marker, both D10 cell fractions were separated from each other with FACSVantage® Cell Sorter and their gene expression was analysed comparatively by using human GeneChip®-based genome-wide gene expression profiling. Four GeneChips® Human Genome U133A 2.0 expression arrays (Affymetrix, UK Ltd.) were used for gene expression profiling (**FIGURE 9 B**). Briefly, subconfluent D10 cells of three 150cm^2 tissue culture flasks (TPP, MIDSCI, Saint Louis, France) were detached with 0.05% trypsin with 0.01% EDTA and counted with trypan blue (Sigma-Aldrich, Steinheim, Germany). About 40x10^6 D10 cells were isolated and centrifuged at 1400rpm for 5min. After the supernatant was removed, the pellet was resuspended in 25μl PBS containing 2% FBS for 1x10^6 cells. Afterwards, D10 cells were labelled with 2.5μl fluorochrome-linked monoclonal antibodies against CD133 (CD133/2PE, Miltenyi Biotech) for 1x10^6 cells. Following 30min of antibody incubation in the dark at 4°C, D10 cells were washed twice with PBS, containing 2% FBS. Subsequently, D10 cells were resuspended in 5ml polyethylene tubes (BD Falcon™, BD Biosciences, San Jose, CA, USA) at a concentration of 10^7 cells/ml in a sorting solution. To avoid cells from sticking to the tube's inner surface, 5ml polyethylene tubes were coated with 1% BSA, and in order to maintain single cell suspension and prevent cell clumping, the sorting solution based on PBS, contained 0.5% BSA and 5mM EDTA. CD133+ and CD133- D10 cells were sorted out in duplicate by FACSVantage® cell sorter until 10^6 cells of each condition were collected in cDMEM in uncoated polyethylene 5ml tubes (BD, Falcon). The results of the cell sorting are shown in **FIGURE 4** and **FIGURE 5**.

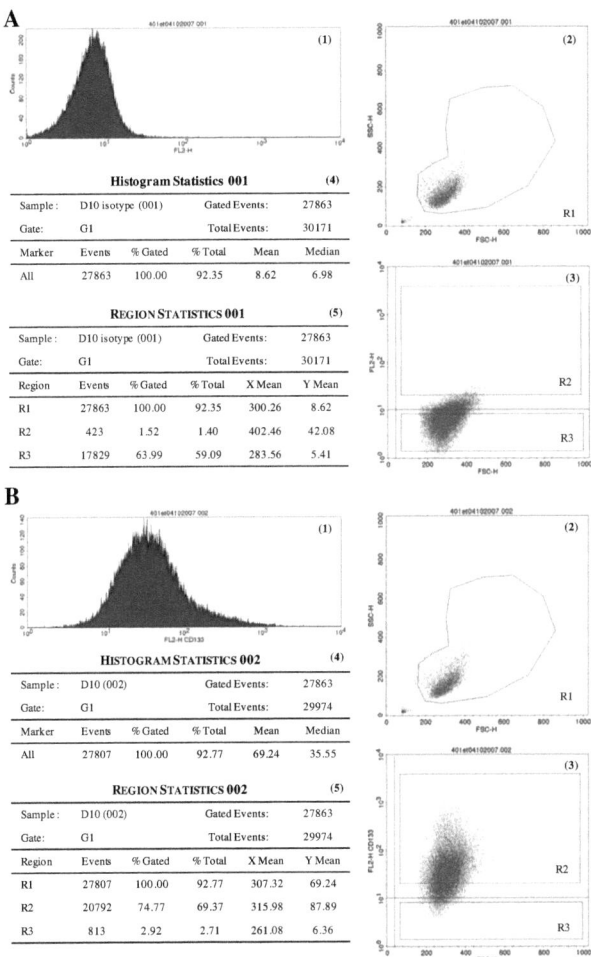

FIGURE 4 A Results of flow cytometric analysis (FACS) before the actual cell sorting. Histogram (1) and dotplots (2) + (3) of D10 cells, incubated with a monoclonal mouse IgG (Isotype control). Corresponding Histogram and dotplot statistics to graphs of the negative control are displayed in the tables (4) and (5). **B** flow cytometry analysis of CD133 expression in D10. In 4% formaldehyd fixed cells were incubated with anti-CD133 (epitope 2, CD133/2).Histogram (1) and dotplots (2) + (3) of D10 cells, labeled with anti CD133 PE–conjugated monoclonal antibody. More than 90% of gated D10 cells express CD133. Region R2 (69.4%) includes CD133+ cells selected to be sorted by FACS Vantage.Corresponding Histogram and dotplot statistics to the graphs are displayed in the tables (4) and (5).

Materials And Methods

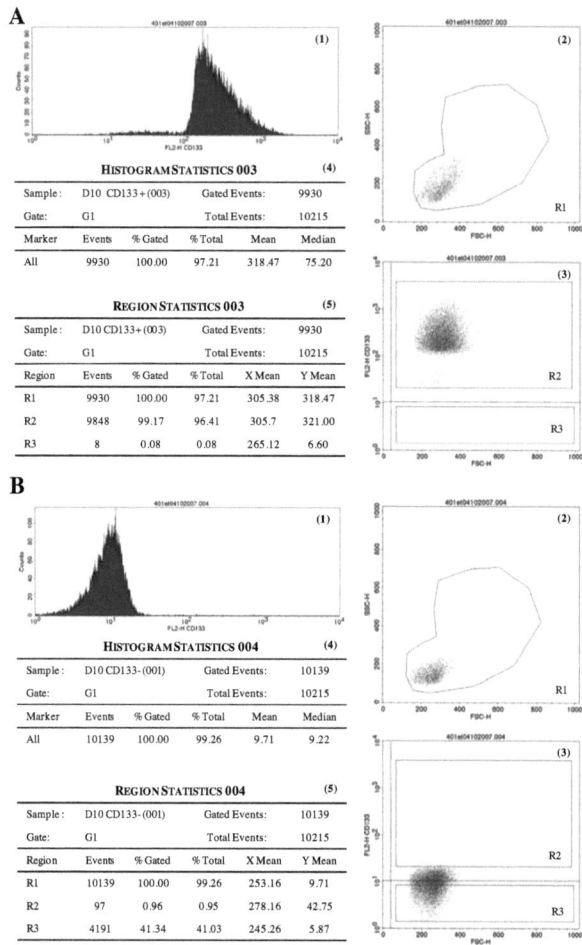

FIGURE 5 A Results of Fluorescent-Activated-Cell-Sorting (FACS) by FACS Vantage. Histogram (1) and dotplots (2) + (3) of sorted CD133+ D10 cells. The fraction of D10 cells positively sorted for CD133 includes more than 97-99% of gated cells (Region R2). Corresponding Histogram and dotplot statistics to the graphs are displayed in the tables (4) and (5). **B** Results of Fluorescent-Activated-Cell-Sorting (FACS) by FACS Vantage. Histogram (1) and dotplots (2) + (3) of sorted CD133- D10 cells. The fraction of CD133- sorted cells includes almost 42% of gated cells (Region R3). Corresponding Histogram and dotplot statistics to the graphs are displayed in the tables (4) and (5).

RNA PREPARATION FOR TARGET SYNTHESIS

FIGURE 6 summarizes the target synthesis protocol starting from total RNA isolation.

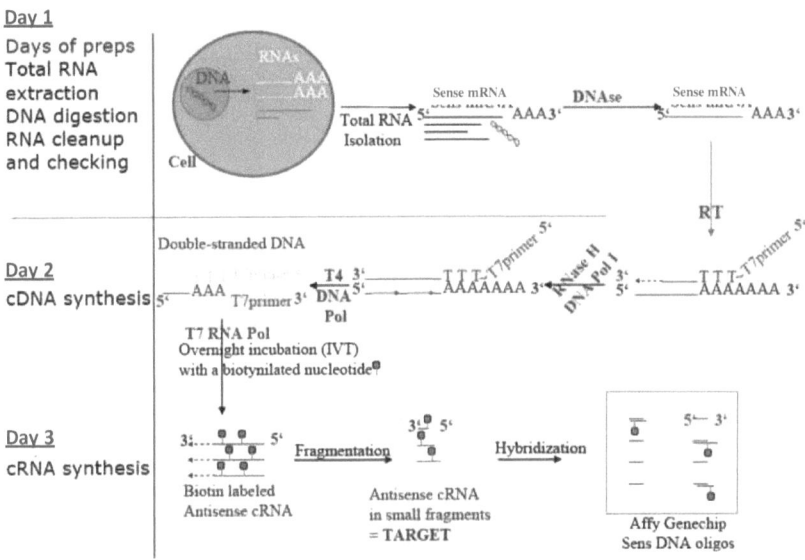

FIGURE 6 Protocol of the gene expression profiling experiments using Affymetrix® GeneChips®. The protocol includes RNA preparation (RNA extraction, DNA digestion, RNA cleanup and checking), target synthesis (cDNA synthesis, cRNA synthesis, Fragmentation) and hybridization of the target onto the GeneChip®. Review **D SUPPLEMENTARY MATERIAL; DETAILED PROTOCOL OF TARGET SYNTHESIS** for further information about the protocol.

TOTAL RNA ISOLATION

Total RNA isolation was carried out using RNeasy Mini Kit (Qiagen, Basel, Switzerland). The four samples of 1×10^6 sorted cells each were disrupted by adding $600 \mu l$ RLT Lysis Buffer (Qiagen), supplemented with 1% β-Mercaptoethanol (Sigma-Aldrich, Steinheim, Germany). In order to obtain a clear and homogenous lysate, the cell pellet was loosened thoroughly by mixing, vortexing and flicking the tubes. Subsequently, the homogenized lysate was centrifuged at 14.000rpm for 2 min. The supernatant was then transferred to new RNase-free tubes and stored frozen at -20°C.

The following procedures were carried out in the laboratories of the Life Science Training Facility (LSTF) of the Biozentrum (Basel, Switzerland) as outlined in **FIGURE 6**.

RNA BINDING TO THE COLUMN
The volume of each lysate was measured with a micropipette and mixed with the same volume of 70% ethanol. $600 \mu l$ of the mixture were applied onto an RNeasy Mini-column, and centrifuged at 12.000rpm for 20s. The flow-through was discarded. The columns were reloaded with the remaining volume of the mixture, centrifuged again at 12.000rpm for 20s and the flow-through was discarded.

COLUMN WASHING
RNeasy columns were washed with $350 \mu l$ Buffer RW1, centrifuged at 12.000rpm for 20s and $80 \mu l$ of DNAse solution were applied to each column and incubated for 15min. Following incubation, RNeasy columns were washed again with $350 \mu l$ Buffer RW1 at same speed and time and the flow-through was discarded. RNeasy columns were transferred onto new 2ml collection tubes and washed with $500 \mu l$ of Buffer RPE at same speed and time. Another $500 \mu l$ of Buffer RPE were pipetted onto the columns and centrifuged at 12.000rpm for 2 minutes to dry the RNeasy silica-gel membrane. The flow-through was discarded and the RNeasy columns were centrifuged again at 14.000rpm for 60s to ensured dryness of the columns.

RNA ELUTION
RNeasy columns were transferred onto RNAse-free 1.5ml tubes and $50 \mu l$ of RNAse-free water were deposited onto the middle of the column matrix. After 1 minute of incubation, columns were centrifuged at 14.000rpm for 60s. The elution step was repeated again. The flow-through of 100µl contained eluted RNA.

RNA CLEANUP
RNA cleanup was performed using RNeasy®MinElute® Cleanup Kit (50), Cat# 74204)). 350µl Buffer RLT and 250µl 100% ethanol was mixed by pipetting with 100µl eluted RNA. The sample, now containing 700µl, was transferred to an RNeasy MinElute spin column placed in a supplied 2ml collection tube. The lid was closed gently and the sample was

centrifuged for 15s at 10.000rpm. The flow-through was discarded. The RNeasy® MinElute® spin column was placed in a new supplied collection tube and 500µl Buffer RPE was pipetted to the spin column. Again, the sample was centrifuged for 15s at 10.000rpm to wash the spin column membrane and the flow-through was discarded. Finally, 500µl of 80% ethanol were added to the RNeasy® MinElute® spin column and centrifuged for 2min at 10.000rpm to wash the spin column membrane. Both flow-through and collection tube were discarded. The RNeasy® MinElute® spin column was placed open-lidded in a new 2ml supplied collection tube for centrifugation at full speed for 5min. Flow-through and collection tube were discarded again. The last step of RNA cleanup included a final washing procedure using 14µl RNase-free water directly placed to the center of the spin column membrane of the spin column in a new 1.5ml collection tube. In order to elute the RNA samples were centrifuged for 1min at full speed.

RNA QUANTIFICATION USING NANODROP®

RNA yield was quantified by spectrophotometric analysis (NanoDrop® Technologies, Wilmington, USA) using the convention that 1 absorbance unit at 260 nm equals to 40 µg/ml RNA. The absorbance was checked at 260 and 280 nm for determination of sample concentration and purity. The A260/A280 ratio should be close to 2.0 for pure RNA (ratios between 1.9 and 2.1 are acceptable). Integrity of total RNA samples was assessed qualitatively on an Agilent 2100 Bioanalyzer®.

RNA VERIFICATION USING BIOANALYZER AGILENT 2100®

Aliquots of each sample were saved for RNA fragment analysis using RNA 6000 Nano Kit (Agilent Technologies, Basel, Switzerland), including RNA chips containing an interconnected set of micro channels that are used for separation of nucleic acid fragments based on their size as they are driven through it electrophoretically. **FIGURE 7** shows the results of 18s and 28s RNA fragments examined on an Agilent 2100 Bioanalyzer (Agilent Technologies, Basel, Switzerland) as follows:

After a new RNA 6000 Nano Chip® was put on the priming station, 9μl gel-dye mix was pipetted in the well marked "G" and the priming station was closed

Materials And Methods 35

(http://cat.ucsf.edu/pdfs/Nano_RNA_Analysis.pdf). The plunger of the priming station was pressed until it was held by the clip. Following exactly 30s the clip was released and 9µl gel-dye mix was applied in the well marked "G". All 12 sample wells and the well for the ladder were loaded with 5µl Agilent RNA 6000 Nano Marker. The previously prepared ladder was applied to the ladder well and the sample wells were loaded with 1µl of sample. All unused sample wells were loaded with 1µl RNA 6000 Nano marker and the chip was vortexed horizontally for 1min at 2400rpm in the adapter. Finally, the chip was inserted into the Bioanalyzer and fragment size of ribosomal RNA for 18s and 28s was examined (**FIGURE 7**).

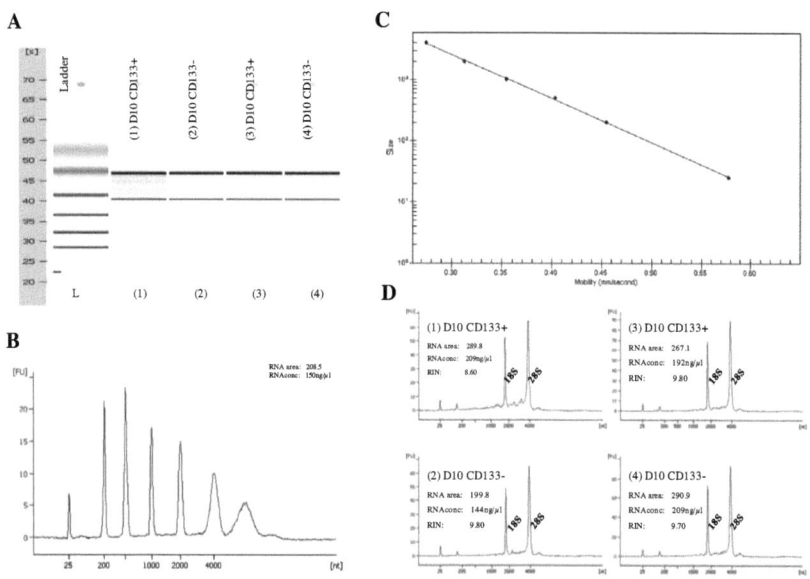

FIGURE 7 Electrophoresis Run Summary. Verification of total RNA isolated from the D10 duplicates, CD133+ [samples (1) + (3)] and CD133- [samples (2) + (4)]. **A** agarose gel, **B** results for ladder (L), **C** standard curve, **D** sample electropherograms use to train RIN. [FU] = fluorescence , [s] = seconds, [nt] = number of nucleotides, RIN = RNA integrity number . The RIN software algorithm (Agilent Technologies) allows for the classification of eukaryotic total RNA, based on a numbering system from 1 to 10, with 10 being the most intact RNA profile.

TARGET SYNTHESIS

Biotin labelling of RNA was performed as described in the GeneChip® Expression Analysis Technical Manual (Affymetrix, Santa Clara, USA). Double-stranded cDNA was synthesized according to the One-Cycle cDNA Synthesis Kit (Affymetrix, Cat# 900431), starting from 5 µg of total RNA. The material was purified with the Sample Cleanup Module (Affymetrix, Cat# 900371).

The purified cDNA was used for an in vitro transcription reaction by using the IVT labelling kit (Affymetrix, Cat# 900449) to synthesize cRNA in the presence of a biotin-conjugated ribonucleotide analog. Labelled cRNA from each reaction was purified by using the Sample Cleanup Module, and average size of the cRNA molecules was assessed on RNA Nano 6000 Chips using Agilent Bioanalyzer 2100. The cRNA targets were incubated at 94°C for 35 min in the provided fragmentation buffer and the resulting fragments of 50–150 nucleotides were again monitored using the Bioanalyzer (**FIGURE 8**). All synthesis reactions were carried out using a PCR machine (T1 Thermocycler; Biometra, Göttingen, Germany) to ensure the highest possible degree of temperature control. The hybridization cocktail (130µl) containing fragmented biotin-labelled target cRNA at a final concentration of 0.05µg/µl was transferred into Affymetrix Human Genome U133A 2.0 and incubated at 45°C on a rotator in a hybridization oven 640 (Affymetrix) for 16 h at 60 rpm. The arrays were washed and stained on a Fluidics Station 450 (Affymetrix) by using the Hybridization Wash and Stain Kit (Affymetrix, Cat# 900720). In order to increase the signal strength the antibody amplification protocol (FS450_0002) was used. The gene chips were processed with an Affymetrix GeneChip® Scanner 3000 7G (Affymetrix) DAT image files of the microarrays were generated using GeneChip Operating Software (GCOS 1.4; Affymetrix). These procedures are explained in **FIGURE 6** and **FIGURE 9** and the following chapter.

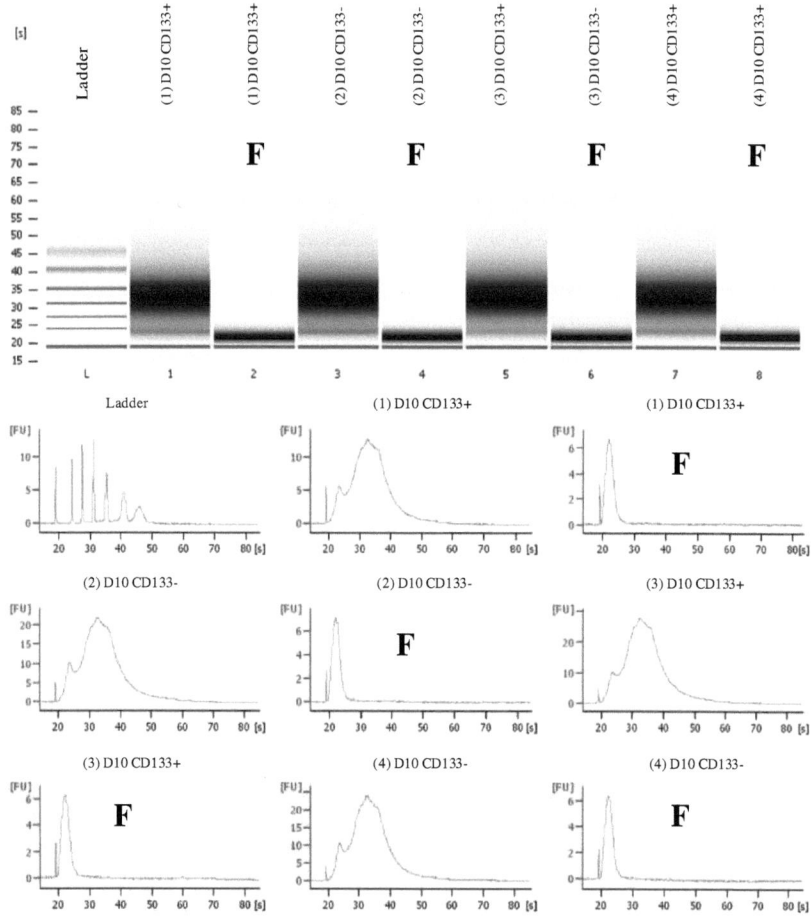

FIGURE 8 Electrophoresis run summary. Verification of cRNA upon fragmentation for target synthesis. Unfragmented (1, 3, 5, 7) and corresponding fragmented (F) samples (2, 4, 6, 8) of cRNA from CD133+ and CD133- D10 cells, respectively. (L) = ladder, (F) = fragmented cRNA samples, [FU] = fluorescence, [s] = seconds.

Materials And Methods 38

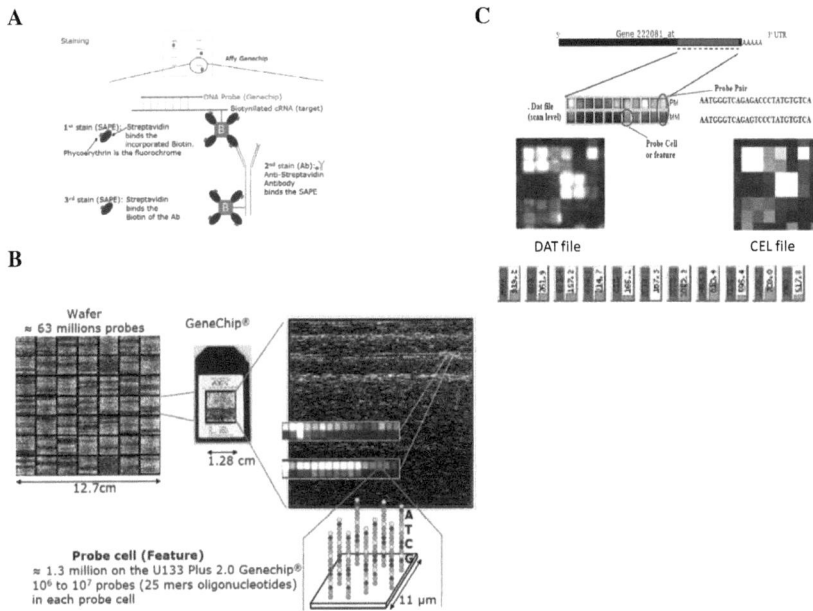

FIGURE 9 A Staining of the probe arrays **B** Affymetrix GeneChip **C** Probe cell distribution. Each gene on the Affymetrix® GeneChip® is represented by a probe set. Each probe set consists of 11-20 probe pairs of oligonucleotides with a length of 25. A probe pair consists of perfect match (PM) and mismatch (MM). Probes that are complementary to the sequence of interest are called perfect match (PM), probes that are complementary to the sequence of interest except for homomeric base change (A-T or G-C) at the 13th position are called mismatch (MM). MM is created by changing the middle (13th) base, to measure non-specific binding.

RESULTS

CHARACTERIZATION OF MELANOMA CELL LINES

INTRODUCTION

Recent evidence suggests that a subset of cells within a tumour have 'stem-like' characteristics. These tumour-initiating cells (TICs), distinct from non-malignant stem cells, show low proliferative rates, high self-renewing capacity, propensity to differentiate into actively proliferating tumour cells, resistance to chemotherapy or irradiation. They are often characterized by elevated expression of stem cell surface markers, in particular CD133 [Neuzil et al. 2007], and sets of differentially expressed genes including genes providing information about the state of differentiation and development and the differentiation capacity of cells of interest.

EXPRESSION OF TUMOUR-ASSOCIATED ANTIGENS

A panel of melanoma cell lines, representative of tumours at diverse differentiation stages was selected. All cell lines derived originally from metastatic melanomas. WM115 cell line was obtained from ATCC; MZ2 cell line was a gift of Dr. van der Bruggen (Brussels, Belgium), whereas HBL, Na8 and D10 were provided by Dr. Eberle (Basel, Switzerland). RE, Me39, Me59 and Me67 cell lines were generated by our group. The expression of a panel of melanoma-associated antigens (MAA) was used to characterize the cell lines under investigation. The antigens under investigation belong to two main groups: tumour-associated cancer/testis- antigens (CTA) including MAGE-A, BAGE, GAGE, NY-ESO-1 and PRAME families and melanoma differentiation antigens. The latter group, including melanosomal matrix protein (gp100), melanoma antigen recognized by T cells (Melan-A/MART-1) and tyrosinase, a key enzyme in biosynthesis of melanin, comprises proteins involved in melanogenesis. These genes are also expressed in non-transformed melanocytes. In contrast, CTA are expressed in several malignancies of different histological origin and are also expressed on a few non-neoplastic cell populations including spermatogonia and throphoblast, but not in healthy melanocytes. The melanoma antigen-A-3 (MAGE-A3) and NY-ESO-1 were selected as representative of the CTA group [Vaughan et al. 2004]. In this study the panel of cell lines was investigated to evaluate their repertoire of melanoma-associated antigens (MAA) partially reflecting specific differentiation stages. Interestingly, HBL and D10 cells expressed melanoma differentiation antigens whereas MZ2, RE, Me59 and Me67 cell lines rather expressed CTA of the MAGE-family. Na8 cell lines neither expressed melanoma differentiation markers nor CTA (**TABLE 4**).

TABLE 4   EXPRESSION OF MAA* IN MELANOMA CELL LINES

	Melanoma differentiation antigens			Cancer/testis antigens	
	Gene expression			Gene expression	
Cell line	gp100	tyrosinase	MART-1	*MAGE 3*	*NY-ESO*
D10	+	+	++	++	-
WM115		+		++	-
HBL	+	+	++	++	-
Na8	-	-	-	-	-
MZ2	-	-	-	++	-
Me59	-	-	-	+/-	
Me67	-	-	-	++	-
RE	-	-	-	++	-
Me39	-	-	++	++	-

*MAA = melanoma-associated antigens; Expression levels were assessed using conventional PCR and evaluated semiquantitatively by densitometry. **Gp100** = melanosomal matrix protein gp100 ; **tyrosinase** = key enzyme in melanin biosynthesis; **MART-1** = Melan/MART-1 = melanoma antigen recognized by T cells; **MAGE3** = melanoma antigen-A3 family, **NY-ESO** = cancer/testis antigen (see text); (+) = moderate expression; (++) = strong expression; (-) = no expression detectable.

EXPRESSION OF GENES ASSOCIATED WITH STEMNESS IN MELANOMA CELL LINES

Embryonic stem cells (ES) are pluripotent cells with indefinite replication potential, exhibiting unlimited multilineage differentiation capacity and plasticity. Fundamental pathways and networks to self-renewal and differentiation have been identified in ES and found to be of relevance in TIC as well. A core group of regulatory genes includes those encoding NANOG, OCT4 and SOX2 transcription factors. Functionally, NANOG cooperates with the other key pluripotent transcription factors OCT4 and SOX2 to control the expression of a set of target genes endowed with important functions in self-renewal and differentiation and limiting each other's expression levels, thereby maintaining ES [Sun et al. 2006; Pan, Thomson 2007]. **NANOG**, a homeodomain transcription factor, is known to be expressed in particular in undifferentiated embryonic stem cells [Yasuda et al. 2006]. It has been shown to be essential in the maintenance of pluripotency [Hart et al. 2004; Pan, Thomson 2007] and self-renewal capacity in murine ES and its overexpression retains ES in undifferentiated stages. Hyslop's group [Hyslop et al. 2005] hypothesized that NANOG would act as a gatekeeper of pluripotency in human embryonic stem and carcinoma cells by preventing their differentiation to extraembryonic endoderm and trophectoderm lineages. In the panel of melanoma cell lines under investigation, NANOG was the most frequently expressed transcription factor of this group. In particular, it was strongly expressed in D10, Me39 and RE cells (**TABLE 5**). On the other hand, WM115, Me67 and HBL expressed NANOG at lower levels, whereas in MZ2, Me59 and Na8 cells, NANOG gene expression was virtually undetectable. **OCT4**, a POU-domain transcription factor encoded by the POU5F1 gene, is involved in the maintenance and differentiation of ES, germ cells and pluripotent cells during normal development. Similarly to NANOG, OCT4 is not expressed in differentiated somatic cell types. Notably, however, specific gene expression has been detected in testicular germ cell tumours, including seminoma and embryonal carcinoma [Looijenga et al. 2003; Cheng et al. 2007a; Cheng et al. 2007b] and other tumour cells [Ruangpratheep et al. 2005]. OCT4 gene was highly expressed in Me39 and RE cells. Lower expression levels could be detected in D10, WM115 and Me59 cells as well. All other cell lines failed to express OCT4 gene (**TABLE 5**). **SOX2** SRY (sex determining region Y)-box 2 is an intronless gene encoding a member of the SRY-related HMG-box (SOX) family of transcription factors which are essential for embryonic development and play critical roles in cell fate determination , differentiation and proliferation [Otsubo et al. 2008; Loh et al. 2008]. It is linked together with OCT4 and NANOG in a pluripotent regulatory network [Fong et al. 2008]. SOX2 is frequently down-regulated in gastric cancers and inhibits cell growth through cell-cycle arrest and apoptosis [Otsubo et al. 2008]. The product of this gene is required for stem-cell self-renewal and maintenance in the central nervous system [Shi et al. 2008]. Mutations in this gene have been associated with optic nerve hypoplasia and with syndromic microphthalmia, a severe form of structural eye malformation [Schneider et al. 2008]. This gene lies within an intron of another gene called SOX2 overlapping transcript (SOX2OT). SOX2 was only expressed in WM115 cells. Thus, this was indeed the only cell line of this panel expressing to similar extents NANOG, OCT4 and SOX2 genes (**TABLE 5**).

TABLE 5   EXPRESSION OF REGULATORY CORE TF* IN MELANOMA CELL LINES

Cell line	Transcription factors		
	NANOG	OCT4	SOX2
MZ2	-	-	-
D10	+ +	+	-
Me39	+ +	+ +	-
WM115	+	+	+
RE	+ +	+ +	-
Me59	-	+	-
Me67	+	-	-
Na8	-	-	-
HBL	+	-	-

*TF = transcription factors; **NANOG** = Nanog homeobox; **OCT4** = POU-domain transcription factor; **SOX2** = SRY (sex determining region Y)-box2; (-) = <10E-03; (+) = $\geq$ 10E-03 < 10E-02; (++) = $\geq$ 10E-02. Expression level of TFgene reported as 2^{-Ct}, where Ct = [Ct (TFgene) – Ct (ACTB)]sample.

HOX GENE EXPRESSION

HOX genes were first described in *Drosophila* for their ability to cause segmental homeotic transformations of the body plan [Lewis 1978] and have since been found to be conserved throughout vertebrate evolution, suggesting their importance in patterning the vertebrate body plan. Whereas flies have eight Hox genes located in a single cluster, mammals have 39 HOX genes arranged in four clusters (HOXA-D), which are further subdivided into thirteen paralogous groups based on sequence similarity and position within the cluster [McIntyre et al. 2007] (**FIGURE 10**).

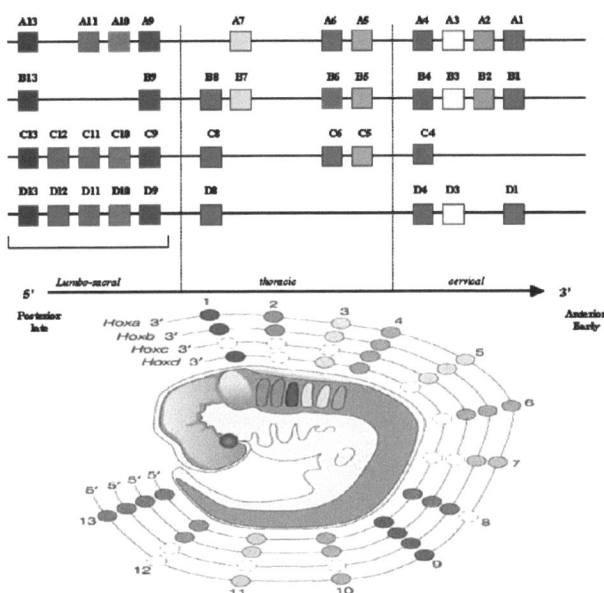

FIGURE 10 HOX gene organization and embryogenesis. The 39 human HOX genes are clustered in four genomci loci, the HOXA, -B, -C. -D complexes, which are further subdivided into thirteen paralogous groups based on sequence similarity and position within the cluster. Horizontal lines represent the four different chromosomes in the upper drawing. Each gene is represented by a colored box. The successive antero-posterior expression domains of HOX genes are schematized in a murine embryo (lower drawing) that has been coloured in the schematic to indicate the approximate domains of transcription expression for all HOX genes. HOX expression along the vertebrate anterior-posterior axis exhibits overlapping expression domains with unique and increasingly posterior limits of expression.

HOX genes are characterized by a conserved 180-bp DNA sequence, the homeobox, coding for a 60-aminoacid DNA-binding domain called the homeodomain. Homeobox genes function as transcription factors [Rubin et al. 1987] recognizing specific DNA sequences and regulate target genes [McGinnis, Krumlauf 1992]. The existence of a vertebrate 'Hox code' that would assign morphologies to each vertebra as a result of the combination of the HOX genes functioning in each region [Kessel, Gruss 1990, Kessel, Gruss 1991, Gruss, Kessel 1991] and meaning that particular sets of paralogous genes provide segmental identity along the anterior-posterior axis of the body has been proposed. This hypothesis could be validated by gene targeting (loss-of-function mutants) or knockout experiments, comparative anatomy studies and the retinoic acid teratogenesis. The 'anterior' HOX genes control the morphogenetic programme of specific hindbrain segments (rhombomeres) or pharyngeal arch neural crest derivatives. In addition, 'posterior' HOXA and HOXD genes act co-ordinately to control the growth and morphogenesis of skeletal structures along the proximo–distal axis of developing limbs [Favier, Dollé 1997].

HOX genes are also expressed in normal adult cells, potentially in a tissue-specific manner involving maintenance of the normal phenotype. In selected malignancies, however, a mis-expression of many HOX genes has been shown [Cillo et al. 1992; Cillo et al. 1999; de Vita et al. 1993; Calvo, Drabkin 2000; Zhu et al. 2002; Cantile et al. 2003], suggesting a possible involvement in carcinogenesis and metastasis. In melanoma cell lines, Svingen [Svingen, Tonissen] could demonstrate an altered HOX gene expression compared to healthy human skin. Maeda and colleagues [Maeda et al. 2005] supported the hypothesis suggesting that aberrant expression of HOX genes was associated with development and subsequent progression of melanoma. However, unlike with fibroblasts [Chang et al. 2002] it could not be shown that the 39 HOX gene expression pattern determines the sites where melanoma grew and thus acts as a postal code of tumour. Furthermore, Morgan et al. [Morgan et al. 2007] demonstrated that the antagonism of HOX/PBX dimer formation blocked the *in vivo* proliferation of melanoma. Taken together, these results suggest that targeting the interaction between HOX and PBX could be selective for the malignant phenotype, in a way that direct knockout of HOX genes would not. Through several publications, Caré's group [Carè et al.

2001; Caré et al. 1996] could show that the HOXB7 gene was functionally associated with melanoma growth promotion through the direct transactivation of bFGF.

HOX gene expression in the nine melanoma cell lines included in our panel was assessed using conventional and quantitative real-time RT-PCR (◆**MATERIALS AND METHODS**). The expression of the four HOX loci using conventional PCR is shown in **FIGURE 11** and the distribution of HOX gene expression among the cell lines investigated is summarized in **FIGURE 12**. Eleven out of 39 HOX genes, which were expressed in all cell lines investigated, were selected and quantitative real-time RT-PCR was performed on these samples. **TABLE 6** shows the mean ΔCt values obtained from the triplicate reactions of the selected 11 HOX genes. It is to be noted that these values reflect exponential amplification and higher ΔCt values represent lower expression. **FIGURE 13/14** also give the results of the quantitative real-time RT-PCR performed on the HOX gene selection but by means of n-fold mRNA expression relative to the calibrator sample (highest ΔCt value), representing the unitary amount of target of interest (◆**MATERIALS AND METHODS**).

Taken together, the collected data indicate that posterior HOXC and HOXD genes are expressed more frequently than anterior HOXA and HOXB genes throughout the panel of melanoma cell lines, in particular, genes of locus HOXC (**FIGURE 11**). Strikingly, 8/9 cell lines, except the cell line HBL, do express more than 70% of locus HOXC genes and 2/3 of all cell lines express more than 70% of HOXD genes. Furthermore, every melanoma cell line expressed all genes of paralogous group 13, including HOXA13, HOXB13, HOXC13 and HOXD13. In addition, the expression of HOXB6, HOXB7, HOXC5, HOXC8-11, HOXD8 and HOXD9 was detectable throughout all cell lines investigated (**FIGURE 12**).

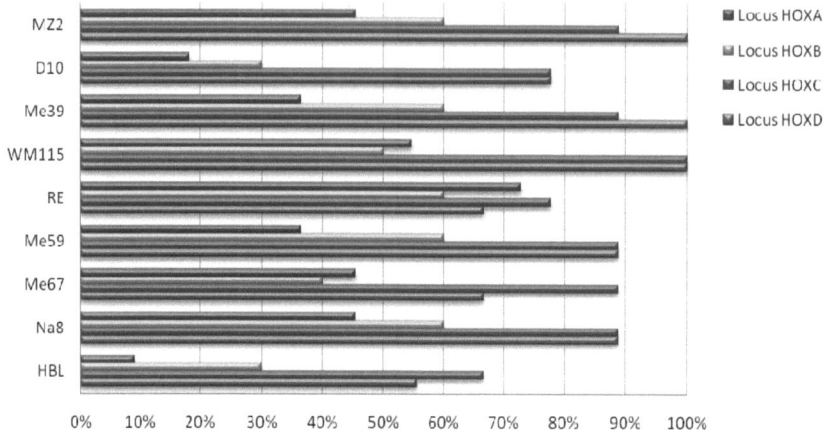

FIGURE 11 Expression of the four HOX loci (HOXA-, -B, -C and –D)in melanoma cells lines. Results of conventional PCR performed on .Each locus is represented by a different colour. The posterior Loci HOXC and HOXD are expressed more frequently in the melanoma cells lines.

The highest expression was detected for HOXC9 and HOXC10 (**TABLE 6**). HOXA13, HOXB7, HOXD9 and HOXD13 were moderately expressed whereas the expression of HOXB13, HOXC8, HOXC11 and HOXC13 was only marginal. The lowest expression was detected for HOXC12. HOXC9 and HOXC10 (SD ± 1.05/1.42) not only were the highest expressed genes but also the most constantly expressed HOX gene across the samples tested whereas the expression of HOXB13 (SD ± 5.24) and HOXD13 (SD ± 3.36) was highly variable. The expression pattern as well as the expression levels of HOXA13 and HOXC13 showed a similar tendency (**TABLE 6, FIGURE 13 A, 14 I**).

HOXD13 expression ranged between three orders of magnitude (**FIGURE 14 L**) whereas the expression levels of all the other HOX genes ranged between one or two orders of magnitude (**FIGURE 13/14, A-K**). Interestingly, the distribution of HOXB7 and HOXD9 as well as HOXC11 and HOXC13 expression among the cell lines seems to be almost equal (**TABLE 6, FIGURE 14 G, I**). While on **FIGURE 12** only WM115 cells expressed HOXC12, the quantitative assay revealed that also D10 and HBL cells do express levels of HOXC12

(**TABLE 6, FIGURE 14 H**) to different extents. HOXB7 expression, published to be associated with melanoma growth, was detectable with subtle differences in all melanoma cell lines considered in this study (**TABLE 6, FIGURE 13 B**). The lowest level of HOXB7 expression was found in HBL cells (calibrator sample) and it was detected to 10 to 60-fold higher extents in the other cell lines.

TABLE 6   QUANTITATIVE RT-PCR ANALYSIS OF HOX EXPRESSION

Gene	MZ2	D10	Me39	WM115	RE	Me59	Me67	Na8	HBL
HOXA13	12,89	8,18	11,88	9,68	np	15,12	9,46	10,99	9,10
HOXB7	10,29	8,57	10,08	7,89	np	9,06	8,53	9,96	13,50
HOXB13	22,64	10,93	12,00	21,35	np	10,58	11,62	10,98	9,00
HOXC8	10,76	12,01	12,39	10,41	np	10,72	18,37	10,38	und
HOXC9	7,00	8,01	9,33	7,62	np	8,43	8,57	6,31	6,59
HOXC10	6,21	5,74	7,55	6,46	np	7,11	5,38	4,54	3,17
HOXC11	11,36	11,46	12,88	11,59	np	15,72	10,55	9,62	11,12
HOXC12	und	19,36	und	12,98	np	und	und	und	14,03
HOXC13	10,16	10,74	13,03	8,98	np	15,67	10,93	10,25	9,33
HOXD9	10,90	9,22	10,71	8,79	np	11,30	10,71	7,84	5,77
HOXD13	7,47	7,97	10,90	9,77	np	10,80	17,62	13,82	8,94

Values represent ΔCt obtained from 11/39 HOX genes in human melanoma cell lines as indicated. Values listed were obtained as described in Materials and Methods, and represent the average ΔCt of individual triplicate reactions; ***np*** = analysis not performed; ***und*** = under level of detection.

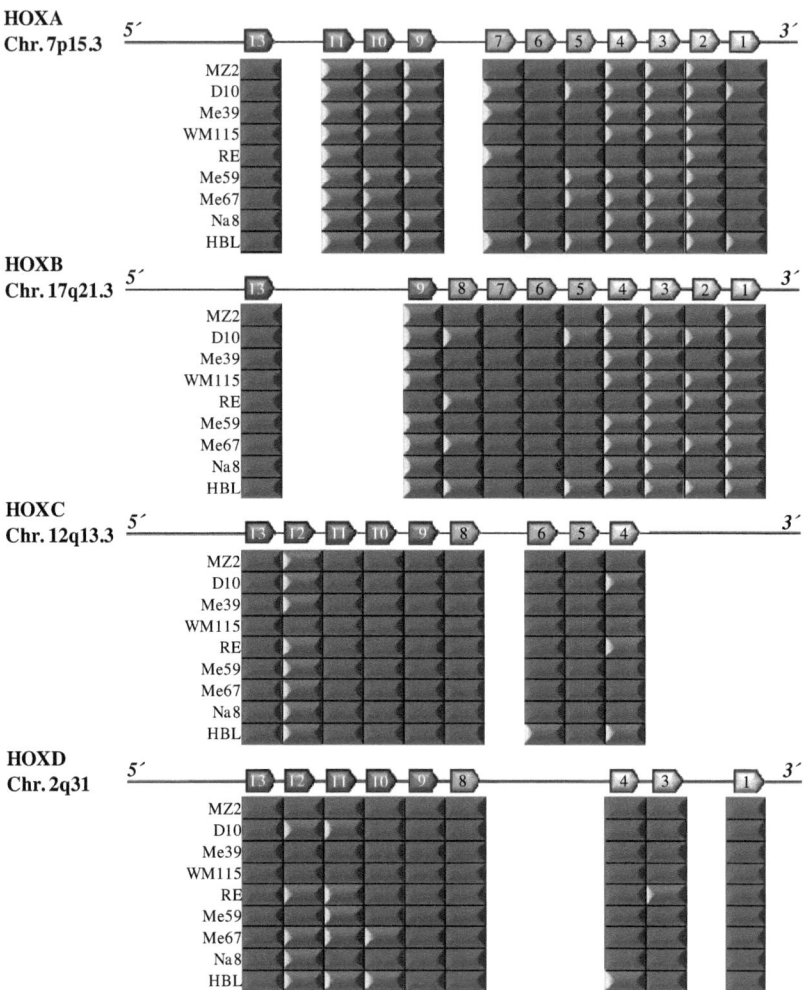

FIGURE 12 HOX gene expression in melanoma cell lines. Results of conventional PCR. Clustered Hox gene organization. The four HOX clusters (HOX A-D) each contain 8–11 genes and are located on four different chromosomes. Each gene is represented by a coloured box. Individual genes in different HOX clusters can be aligned into paralogous groups (identical colours) based on the sequence homology within their homeobox regions. Beyond each HOX cluster the corresponding status of HOX gene expression in melanoma cell lines; red = active gene; blue = inactive gene.

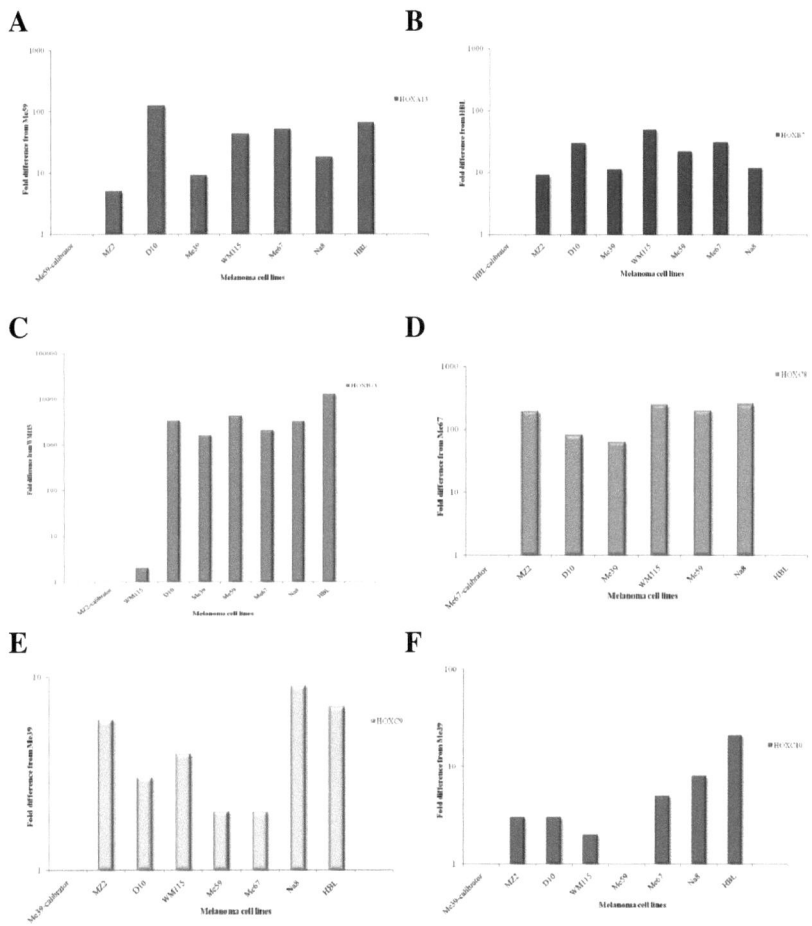

FIGURE 13 Quantitative Real-Time RT-PCR of HOX Expression in Melanoma cell lines. **A** HOXA13; **B** HOXB7; **C** HOXB13; **D** HOXC8; **E** HOXC9; **F** HOXC10. Calibrator sample represents the unitary amount of the target of interest, the other samples express n-fold mRNA relative to the calibrator. Final amounts of target were determined as follows: target amount = 2^{-Ct}, where Ct = [Ct (HOXgene) − Ct (ACTB)]sample − [Ct (HOXgene) − Ct (ACTB)]calibrator.

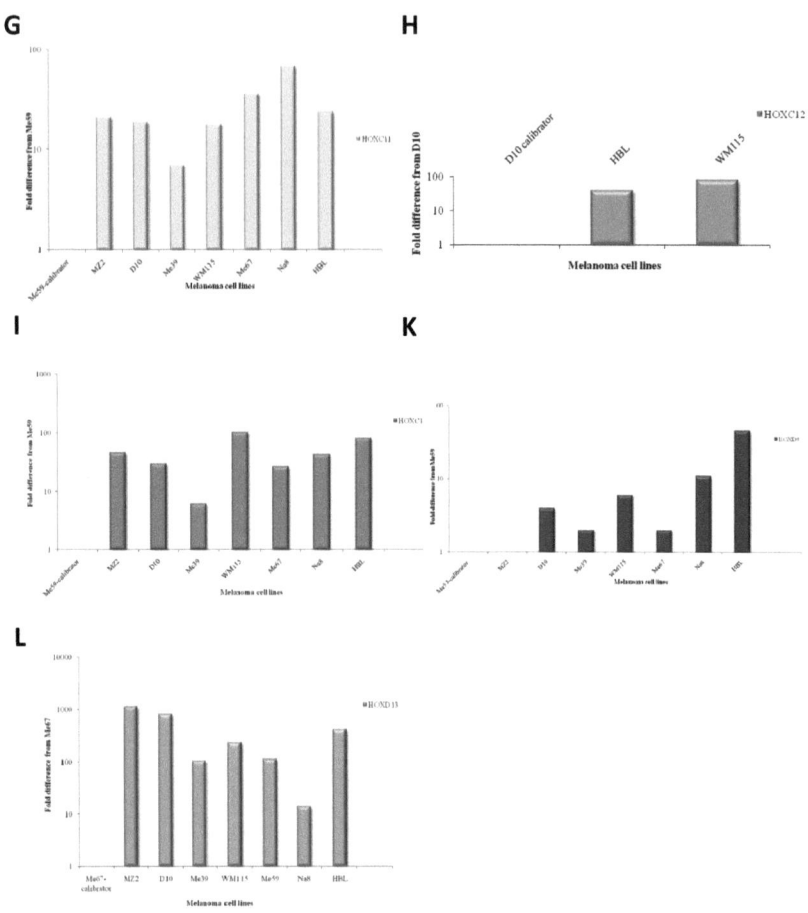

FIGURE 14 Quantitative Real-Time RT-PCR of HOX Expression in Melanoma cell lines. **G** HOXC11; **H** HOXC12; **I** HOXC13; **K** HOXD9; **L** HOXD13. Calibrator sample represents the unitary amount of the target of interest, the other samples express n-fold mRNA relative to the calibrator. Final amounts of target were determined as follows: target amount = 2^{-Ct}, where Ct = [Ct (HOXgene) – Ct (ACTB)]sample – [Ct (HOXgene) – Ct (ACTB)]calibrator.

Phenotypic Characterization Of Melanoma Cell Lines

Selection of surface markers

A number of surface molecules have been reported to be expressed on embryonic stem cells, bone marrow derived mesenchymal stem cells (MSC) with multilineage differentiation capability and on putative cancer stem cells (CSC). Recent data revealed that CD133 is highly expressed in CSC populations from different types of cancers, including medulloblastoma [Singh et al. 2003], glioblastoma [Salmaggi et al. 2006; Liu et al. 2006a], as well as prostate [Collins et al. 2005; Richardson et al. 2004] and colon carcinomas [O'Brien et al. 2007; Ricci-Vitiani et al. 2007]. In particular, Frank´s group [Frank et al. 2005] recently showed that CD133+/ABCG5+ melanoma cells were resistant to doxorubicin treatment and that melanoma tissue isolated from patients expressed high levels of both CD133 and ABCG5. Furthermore, WM115 cell line was reported to contain a CD133+ subpopulation of melanoma cancer cells capable of initiating a tumour upon transplantation into immunocompromised mice [Monzani et al. 2007].

Human CD133 (human prominin-1), a five transmembrane domain glycoprotein, was originally identified as a cell surface antigen present on CD34+ hematopoietic stem cells. Although the biological function of CD133 is not well understood, antibodies to CD133 epitopes have been widely used to purify hematopoietic stem and progenitor cells. Furthermore, a number of non-lymphoid tissues including placenta, kidney, prostate, liver epithelial and endothelial cells as well as neural cells display CD133 expression. Cells expressing CD133 are thought to be responsible for the large capacity of regeneration of these tissues and, accordingly, emerge as stem cells in their specific environment. Interestingly, in cases of mutational transformation, CD133+ stem cells from adult tissues might give rise to malignant cancer stem cells which are still identifiable by their specific phenotype. In these conditions CD133 can also be considered a cancer stem cell marker characterizing a population of cancer cells able to reconstitute a tumour upon transplantation in immunodeficient hosts [Bidlingmaier et al. 2008].

CD117, c-KIT or SCFR (stem cell factor receptor), a glycoprotein of the tyrosine kinase receptor (TKR) family is expressed on stem cells, bone marrow stromal cells, pluripotent hematopoietic progenitor cells, fibroblasts and melanocytes. One of the natural ligands for CD117 is the stem cell growth factor.

The melanoma cell adhesion molecule (MCAM) CD146 is expressed on throphoblast, endothelium and melanoma cells. Since it is also expressed in endothelial cells in highly vascularised tissues, CD146 appears to be associated with tumour progression and metastasis in human melanomas. Haematogenous metastases could be enhanced by the interaction of CD146 with cellular elements of vascular tissue. Thus, CD146 might be particularly useful to stage progression of malignant melanomas.

CD271, belonging to the tumour necrosis factor receptor superfamily, is a low affinity receptor for nerve growth factor (NGF). CD271 (NGFR) is not only expressed on neurons but also on bone marrow mesenchymal cells and melanocytes.

Transforming growth factor ß (TGF-ß) plays key roles in cell differentiation and angiogenesis and it binds to CD105. Thus CD105 (Endoglin, ENG) expression modulates the cellular response to TGF ß which, in turn, regulates cell differentiation and migration of stem cells, endothelial cells, bone marrow stromal cells and mesenchymal cells. The level of CD105 increases in response to TGFß, as demonstrated in cell lines transfected with CD105(...).

EXPRESSION OF SURFACE MARKERS ON MELANOMA CELL LINES

Melanoma cell lines were stained with fluorochrome labelled monoclonal antibodies (mAbs) in order to reveal the expression of the specific markers under investigation. TABLE 7A reports percentages of cells staining positive for the surface markers of interest whereas TABLE 7B indicates the corresponding mean fluorescence intensity (MFI) values which are expressed as differential intensity of the signal emitted by the antibody of interest as compared to the signal provided by the mouse isotype (signal [mAbs] - signal[IgG]).

Our data indicate that melanoma cell lines express discrete stem cell markers. However, the distribution of the expression was highly variable among the cell lines under investigation (TABLE 7A/7B).

TABLE 7A		MELANOMA PHENOTYPE			
Cell line	CD133+	CD105+	CD146+	CD271+	CD117+
MZ2	neg.	86.41	73.92	99.74	neg.
D10	89.66	77.14	98.79	neg.	neg.
Me39	1.88	95.65	100.00	7.40	neg.
WM115	neg.	87.60	99.6	45.24	neg.
RE	3.11	74.84	98.31	59.96	1.28
Me59	1.00	75.55	36.40	2.72	18.95
Me67	neg.	75.94	73.76	10.75	neg.
Na8	1.05	97.22	0.67	82.54	neg.
HBL	neg.	22.66	30.08	2.32	99.46

Expression levels of flourochrome-conjugated monoclonal antibodies against surface markers of interest on melanoma cell lines. Frequency and distribution of cells carrying surface markers expressed as percentages of positive gated cells; neg indicates percentages of positive gated cells < 1%.

TABLE 7B		MELANOMA PHENOTYPE			
Cell line	CD133+	CD105+	CD146+	CD271+	CD117+
MZ2	neg.	16.66	14.01	499.9	neg.
D10	60.14	11.1	342.72	neg.	neg.
Me39	neg.	15.36	206.38	6.47	neg.
WM115	neg.	15.53	355.32	12.53	neg.
RE	neg.	12.45	686.77	14.11	neg.
Me59	neg.	15.69	7.38	neg.	3.95
Me67	neg.	11.21	16.04	1.25	neg.
Na8	neg.	32.81	neg.	51.38	neg.
HBL	neg.	4.46	5.75	neg.	81.83

Single staining. Corresponding intensities of surface marker expression on melanoma cell lines (TABLE 7A). Results displayed as mean fluorescence intensity values (MFI): MFI = signal [mAb] − signal [isotype control]. No signal detected was indicated by (neg.) when MFI < 1.

Over 80% of D10 cells expressed CD133 (**FIGURE 15**). In addition, nearly 2% of Me39 cells, more than 3% of RE cells and more than 1% of Na8 and Me59 cells also expressed CD133.

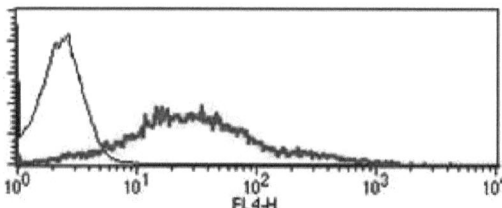

FIGURE 15 Phenotype of D10 cell line. Expression levels of APC-conjugated monoclonal antibodies against the CD133 epitope (red graph).

Strikingly, CD105, the TGF-β receptor was detectable on more than 75% of the cells of all melanoma cell lines under investigation with the exception of HBL. In this cell line only 23% of cells expressed CD105. All Na8 cells were CD105 positive.

CD271, the nerve growth factor receptor (NGFR) was expressed to variable extents in 8/9 cell lines, except on D10 cells. Expression levels ranged between 2% (HBL) and more than 99% (MZ2). Na8 and HBL showed peculiar patterns of CD105, CD271 and CD117 expression. Virtually 83% of Na8 cells bound anti-CD271 antibody as opposed to 2% of HBL cells. In stark contrast, CD117 (c-kit) expression levels displayed an opposite pattern with less than 1% positivity in Na8 cells and more than 99% in HBL. Furthermore, more than 1% of RE cells and almost 19% of Me59 were identified to express CD117. Similarly to CD271, CD146 was also expressed on 8/9 cell lines but Na8 remained the only cell line of this panel which was not expressing CD146. Almost all D10, Me39, WM115 and RE cells expressed CD146 with high MFI. In contrast, although more than 73% of Me67 and MZ2 cells expressed CD146, this surface marker was only detectable at relatively low fluorescence intensity values (MFI between14 and 16). WM115 was previously reported to contain a CD133+ subpopulation. This could not be confirmed in our experiments. Nonetheless, two subpopulations were identified in WM115. One fraction stained positive for CD105 (88%) and another one for CD271 (45%).

In general, HBL emerged as an outstanding cell line in our panel since virtually all cells expressed CD117 with relatively high intensity. No other surface marker under investigation was found to be expressed in these cells under these conditions.

PHENOTYPE UPON 3D-CULTURE

Evidence of the capacity of cancer stem cells to grow in spheroid structures has been repeatedly reported (✦ **INTRODUCTION** and **MATERIALS AND METHODS**). To assess these features in the melanoma cell lines under investigation cell lines were cultured in flasks pre-treated with PolyHEMA, preventing their attachment to the plastic surface. In these conditions, Na8 cell line was clearly generating spheroids (**FIGURE 16**) whereas D10 and HBL grew in aggregates. Thus, phenotypes of these three cell lines were assessed upon 3D culture. Cells were labelled again with monoclonal antibodies (mAbs) against CD133, CD117, CD105, CD271 and CD146 and the results were compared with the stainings observed in cells cultured in 2D. Interestingly, the only modification observed in 3D as compared to 2D cultures was represented by a modest increase of the fraction of CD133+ cells in Na8 cell line. In contrast, expression levels of CD105, CD117, CD146 and CD271 were unmodified (data omitted for simplicity).

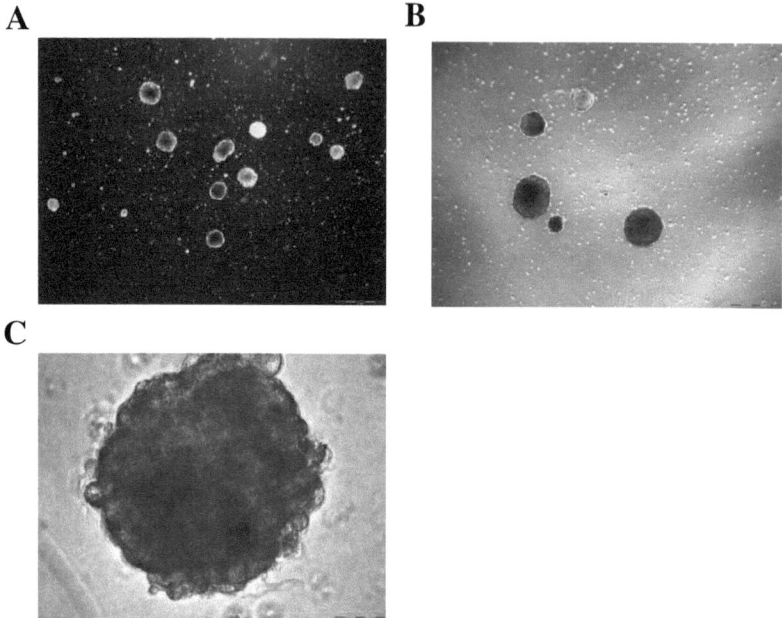

FIGURE 16 Na8 spheroids in polyHEMA-coated tissue culture flask. **A** = 2x magnification, **B** = 4x magnifictaion, **C** = 40x magnification.

FUNCTIONAL CHARACTERIZATION OF DIFFERENT CELL LINES

CLONOGENIC ASSAY AND POISSON´S DISTRIBUTION

Clonogenic assays were performed by limiting dilution analysis (LDA) on cells magnetically sorted according to their expression of selected markers. Frequency of proliferating cells was evaluated by Poisson's distribution (✦ **MATERIALS AND METHODS**). Results of a typical experiment are shown in **FIGURE 3**.

CD271 is a surface marker expressed by a sizeable percentage of cells from MZ2 cell line. A 7% of the CD271+ fraction of MZ2 formed colonies, as compared to 5% of the CD271- fraction. Thus, CD271 expression could not be associated with a higher clonogenic capacity in MZ2 cells.

In D10 cell line the capability of CD133 and CD105 markers to identify cells with high clonogenic potential was investigated. CD133+ D10 cells from cell showed a significantly ($p<0.05$) higher clonogenic capacity as compared to CD133- cells. The Poisson's distribution yielded that 41% of the CD133+ cells were capable of giving rise to cell colonies, as opposed to 6% of the negative fraction. In contrast, CD105+ and CD105- D10 cells, displayed a similar clonogenic potential.

In the Me39cell line, where only 6% of the CD105 expressing cells were capable of forming colonies, the fraction of CD105- cells dominated in terms of clonogenic capacity since all cells were able to form colonies. Both CD271+ and CD271- Me39 cells were comparably poorly capable of forming colonies. WM115 cells expressed CD105 and CD271. The CD105+ fraction showed a significantly higher clonogenic capacity than the CD105- fraction. Almost every third cell of the CD105+ population had the potential to form colonies whereas CD105- cells were unable to do it in our experimental conditions. In contrast, CD271+ and CD271- WM115 cells did not significantly differ in their clonogenic potential in as much as 15% and 13%, respectively, were colony forming cells.

RE cells expressed CD105 and CD271. Both, the CD105+ and the CD105- fraction possessed equal clonogenic capacity. On the other hand, while almost all CD271- RE cells were capable of forming colonies only 10% of CD271+ cells were able to do so.

CD105, CD117and CD271 markers were expressed on Me59 cells. CD105+ cells were indistinguishable from CD105- cells based on their clonogenic capacity (2% and 1%, respectively). In contrast significantly higher clonogenic potential was detectable in CD117- and CD271+ cells, as compared to their CD117+ and CD271- counterparts.

Regarding Me67 melanoma cell line CD105 expression failed to identify a cell subset characterized by a predominant clonogenic capacity.

CD105 and CD271 are expressed on Na8 cells. Interestingly, CD105-cells displayed the highest clonogenic capacity. Furthermore, fractions of Na8 cells expressing or lacking CD271 expression did not differ in their clonogenic potential.

CD117 was expressed on almost all HBL cells. Notably, the absence of CD117 expression was not compatible with in vitro survival of those cells. Referring to Poisson`s distribution, almost all HBL cells expressing CD117, are capable of inducing colony growth. HBL cells also expressed CD105 but all CD105- cells formed colonies as opposed to only 2% of CD105+ cells.

GENE EXPRESSION PROFILING OF CD133+ D10 CELLS

Gene expression profiling on sorted (FACS VANTAGE Cell Sorter) CD133+ D10 cells was carried out using four single Affymetrix GeneChip® Human Genome ((U133A2.0) (HG-U133A2.0)) arrays. Results of the sorting are shown in **FIGURE 4** and **5** (♦ **MATERIALS AND METHODS**). Following chip data processing (♦ **MATERIALS AND METHODS**), profiles of genes significantly (p-value < 0.01) up- or down-regulated (+/- 1.3-fold) in CD133+ D10 cells as compared to CD133- D10 cells were obtained (**TABLE 8 AND TABLE 9**).

The GeneChip® HG-U133A 2.0 (**FIGURE 9**) is a single array comprising 22.000 probe sets and 500.000 distinct oligonucleotides. It represents 18.400 transcripts and variants including 14.500 well-characterized human genes. Sequences used in the design of the array were selected from GenBank®, dbEST, and RefSeq. The sequence clusters were created from the UniGene database (Build 133, April 20, 2001) and they were refined by analysis and comparison with a number of other publicly available databases including the Washington University EST trace repository and the University of California, Santa Cruz Golden-Path human genome database (April 2001 release).

PANTHER CLASSIFICATION SYSTEM

Expression data were analyzed using the PANTHER (**P**rotein **AN**alysis **TH**rough **E**volutionary **R**elationships) Classification System. PANTHER classifies genes using published scientific experimental evidence and evolutionary relationships to predict function even in the absence of direct experimental evidence. Proteins are classified into families and subfamilies of shared function, which are then categorized by molecular function and biological process ontology terms. For a large number of proteins, detailed biochemical interactions in canonical pathways are captured and can be viewed interactively.

Our gene expression data set included 68 up-regulated (**TABLE 8**) and 46 down-regulated (**TABLE 9**) genes in CD133+ as compared to CD133- D10 cells (+/- 1.3 fold, p-value < 0.01).

PANTHER UP-REGULATED GENES

Only 3 out of the 68 up-regulated genes IDs, HJURP, LL22NC03-75B3.6 and DCC1, were not recognized by the system and were excluded as unmapped PANTHER IDs whereas 65 gene IDs could be processed and investigated for their molecular function and the biological processes and canonical pathways they are involved in. **FIGURE 17** and **FIGURE 18** display the results of the analysis with the PANTHER classification systems. The analysis shows that out of the 65 mapped PANTHER IDs genes, the molecular functions of 15 (23%) are still unclassified (**FIGURE 17 A**). Eight genes (12%) encode for two subgroups of cytoskeletal proteins; first, actin binding cytoskeletal proteins (ABLIM1, FHOD3, CSRP2, LIMS2 and PLS1) and, second, the family of the microtubule cytoskeletal proteins (KIF23, KIF2C, KIF15). A group of 6 (9%) up-regulated regulatory molecules includes HRASLS3, the G-Protein modulators RASGRP1 and SERGEF, the G-protein RAB15, the kinase modulator CCNF and the protease inhibitor SERPINF1. Six signalling molecules are organized in three subgroups covering the growth factors PDGFC and IGF1, the peptide hormone ADM and the other signalling molecules ERG, HOMER2 and MGP. Considering the biological process (**FIGURE 17 B**) the 65 up-regulated genes are involved in, strikingly, the process of signal transduction captures 17% (n=11) of the genes. This group of up-regulated genes is subdivided into the processes of cell communication (IGFBP3, PDGFC, CEACAM1, IGF, MGP), cell surface mediated signal transduction (RASGRP1, RRH, HOMER2, LIMS2) and intracellular signalling cascades (RASGRP1). The genes encoding for the signal molecules ERG and HRASLS3 are not further classified. Fifteen percent (n=10) of the up-regulated genes are part of developmental processes including meiosis (KIF2C), ectoderm development (ABLIM1, MICAL2), mesoderm development (CSRP2, MGP) and other developmental processes (ERG, KIF15, ADM, IGF, PDGFC). Cell proliferation and differentiation is regulated by 14% (n=9) of the up-regulated genes (BTG3, GTSE1, ERG, PDGFC, KIF15, CCNF, UBE2C, IGF MAFF). Eight genes (12%) influence the cell cycle at stages of mitosis (CDC2, ESPL1, KIF23, KIF15, AURKA and CCNF) and, in particular, CDC2 and CCNF are, together with UBE2C, responsible for controlling the cell cycle. Furthermore, 5 genes, (8%) modulate cell structure (ABLIM1, GTSE1, KIF15 and PLS1) and affect cell motility (ABLIM1 and LIMS2). Also 5 genes are subordinated to subgroups of immunity and defence processes including detoxification (ABHD6), macrophage-mediated immunity (DDT), stress response (GTSE1), T-cell mediated immunity (IFI30) and other immune and defence processes (CXADR). The products of three genes are involved in the p53 pathway. The biological functions of 13 (20%) of the modulated genes is still unclassified. Four genes (6%) are involved in intracellular protein traffic. Among others (KIF15, RAB15, NUP210), the positive control key molecule CD133 (PROM1) also fulfils unknown protein traffic tasks. Seven genes (11%) are involved in protein and DNA metabolism. Protein modifying genes are CDC2, AURKA and UBE2C. SERPINF1, IFI30 and MARCH3 fulfil proteolytic tasks. EEF1A2 regulates translation. ADCY2 is involved the metabolism of cyclic nucleotides, ENTPD1 and AMPD3 affect the purine metabolism and ERG, MAFF and ZXDC influence the mRNA transcription. Finally, SERGEF has a part in the transport of nucleosides, nucleotides and nucleic acid molecules. Only 3 (5%) of the up-regulated genes (FAM129A, ERG and DENND2D) are associated with oncogenesis. The panel of the 65 up-regulated genes is represented in 32 pathways. Except for the p53 pathway, where three genes (GTSE1, CDC2 and IGFBP3) are involved in, the remaining 31 pathways are only occupied by single gene representatives (data not shown).

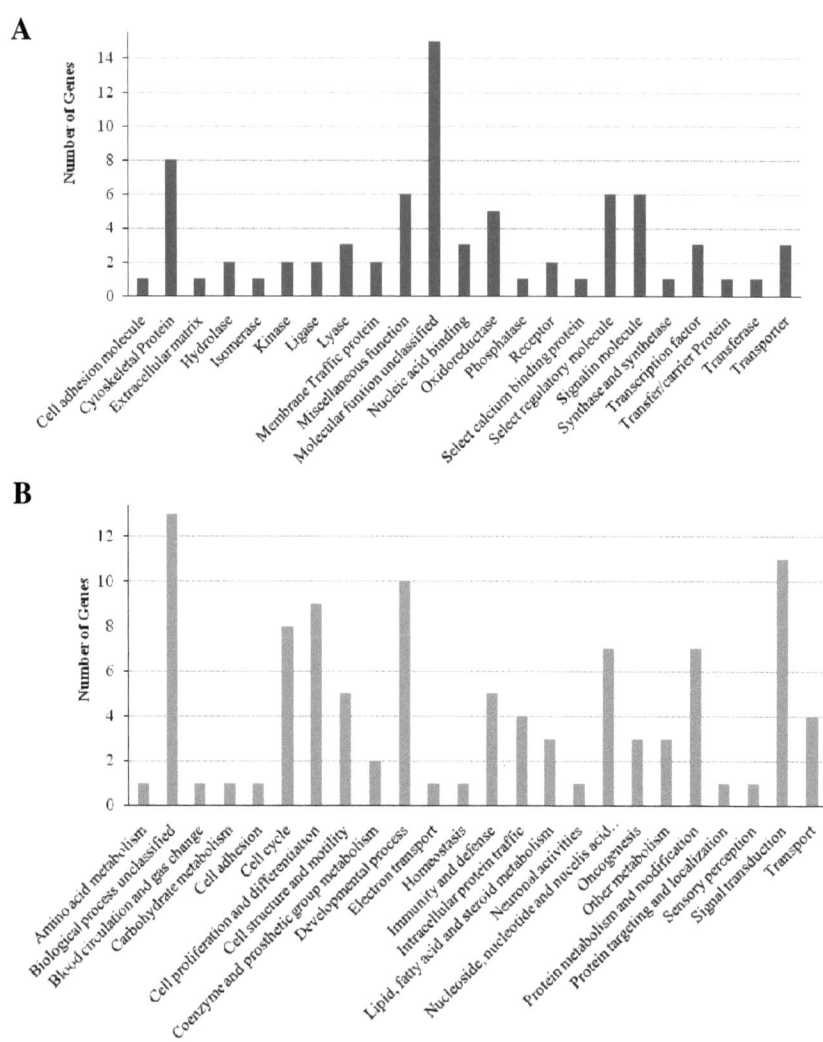

FIGURE 17 Results of PANTHER analysis performed on 65 up-regulated genes in CD133+ D10 cells. Molecular function **A** and biological process **B** those 65 genes are involved in.

PANTHER DOWN-REGULATED GENES

The expression analysis data provide 46 down-regulated genes in CD133+ D10 cells as compared to the CD133- fraction (+/- 1.3 fold, p-value < 0.01). Following the initial gene ID mapping with PANTHER, 44 mapped PANTHER IDs were obtained and analyzed for their molecular functions and the biological processes and pathways they are involved in. The gene symbols GOM1 and CINP could not be recognized by the classification system. Twelve (27%) of the down-regulated genes could not be assigned to a molecular function (**FIGURE 18 A**). Among the remaining genes, 7 (16%) are regulatory molecules including the G-protein modulators RABEPK, CAV1 and RABGEF5, the G-protein RAB40B and the protease inhibitors TIMP1, SPOCK1 and SERPINH1. Four of the down-regulated genes (9%) encode cell adhesion or nucleic acid binding molecules. The group of cell adhesion molecules includes TNC, LSAMP (CAM family), JAM3 and LGALS1, the group of nucleic acid binding proteins includes CITED1, SSX1, EIF4E2 (translation factor) and QKI. Almost one-third of the down-regulated genes (n=14) plays roles in (**FIGURE 18 B**) the transduction of different types of signals. This group includes genes involved in cell communication processes (LEPREL2, STAC, PTPRD, TNC, SLC1A5, SCG2) intracellular signalling cascades (PLK2, STAC, RAB40B, EDNRB, SGK, RAPGEF5) and cell surface receptor mediated signal transduction (CXCR4, CBLB, EDNRB, CAV1). Twenty-five percent (n=11) could not be assigned to a defined biological process and 18% (n=8) are involved in developmental processes including ectoderm development (CXCR4, EDNRB, PTPRD, TNC, LSAMP), embryogenesis (PLK2) and other not further classified developmental processes (EYA2, TIMP1, PTPRD). Seven (16%) down-regulated genes could be assigned to subsets involved in protein metabolism, including protein biosynthesis (EIF4E2), protein modification (PLK2, PTPRD, SGK), proteolysis (TIMP1, SERPINH) and translation regulation (RPL17). The oncogene SSX was down-regulated in CD133+ D10 cells. Two genes of the chemokine- and cytokine-signalling-mediated inflammation pathways (CXCR4 and TNC) and two genes of the integrin pathway (CAV1 and FLNA) were down-regulated in CD133+ D10 cells (data not shown).

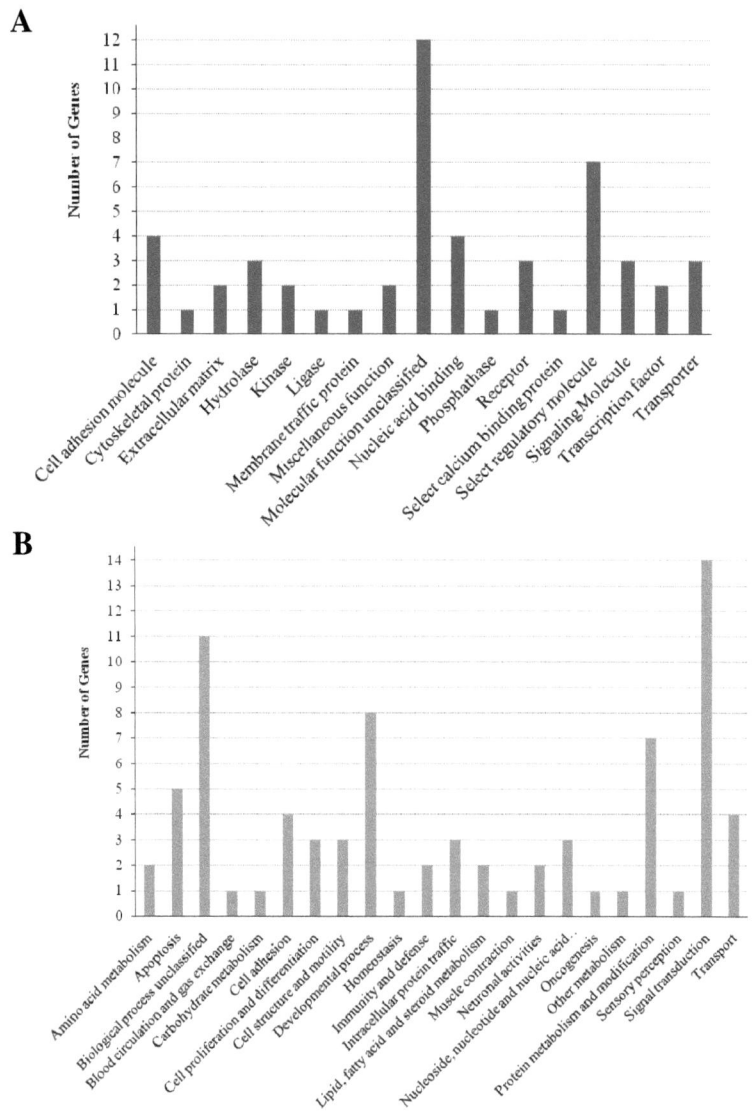

FIGURE 18 Results of PANTHER analysis performed on 44 down-regulated genes in CD133+ D10 cells. Molecular Function **A** and biological process **B** those 44 genes are involved in.

Genes up-regulated more than 2.5-fold (p<0.001) in CD133+, as compared to CD133- D10 cells

The expression of **Matrix GIa Protein** gene (MGP, Matrix Gamma-Carboxyglutamic Acid Protein, MGLAP, NTI; GIG36) was 32-fold up-regulated in CD133+ D10 cells, as compared to CD133- D10 cells. MGP was reported to be expressed at high levels in heart, kidney, and lung and is up-regulated by vitamin D in bone cells. The human genome contains a single copy of the gene. Laize and colleagues [Laizé et al. 2005] showed that MGP is a 10-kD vitamin K-dependent protein produced and secreted by vascular smooth muscle cells and chondrocytes and accumulated in bone, cartilage, and dentin. MGP is a natural inhibitor of calcification and plays important roles in the prevention of vessel calcification and bone differentiation [Yao et al. 2008a; Yao et al. 2008b; Hendig et al. 2008; Schurgers et al. 2007; Gheduzzi et al. 2007; Hermans et al. 2007; Price et al. 1994; Hale et al. 1991; Cancela et al. 1990]. Since Chen et al. [Chen et al. 1990] reported the overexpression of matrix Gla protein mRNA in malignant human breast cells, there has been no further association of MGP with malignancies in general.

The positive control **Prominin 1** (PROM1, RP41; AC133; CD133; PROML1; MSTP061) gene encodes pentaspan transmembrane glycoprotein. CD133 was initially shown to be expressed on primitive hematopoietic stem and progenitor cells and retinoblastoma. CD133 has since been shown to be expressed on hemangioblasts, and neural stem cells as well as on developing epithelium. CD133+ cancer stem cells (CSC) have been identified in haematological malignancies and several solid cancers. Singh [Singh et al. 2003]isolated a CD133+ cell subpopulation from human brain tumours that exhibited stem cell properties in vitro, including a high self-renewal potential and the capability of recapitulating the original tumour in NOD-SCID mice [Singh et al. 2004a; Singh, Dirks 2007; Singh et al. 2004b]. Only the CD133+ brain tumour fraction contained cells that were capable of tumour initiation in NOD-SCID mouse brains. The identification of CD133+ tumour subpopulations was also reported for many other solid tumours (pancreatic cancer, breast cancer) and in malignant melanoma [Frank et al. 2005; Monzani et al. 2007; Klein et al. 2007]. Furthermore, Bao and his group [Bao et al. 2006] showed that CD133+ cancer stem cells contribute to radio resistance through preferential activation of the DNA damage checkpoint response and an increased DNA repair capacity. The fraction of tumour cells expressing CD133is enriched after irradiation in glioma. The expression of CD133 was almost 28-fold up-regulated in CD133+ D10 cells thus confirming the integrity of cell sorting and gene expression profiling.

The **tumour protein D52** gene (TPD52, TPD52-like 1, D52, N8L, PC-1, PrLZ, hD52) is expressed as a 1.5-kb transcript in human kidney, skin, and some breast tumours [Boutros et al. 2004]. The expression of the gene coding for TPD52 was 3.7-fold up-regulated in CD133+ D10 cells. Byrne´s group [Byrne et al. 1996] suggested that TPD52 may be involved in calcium-mediated signal transduction and cell proliferation.

Ectonucleoside triphosphate diphoyphorylase 1 (D) (ENTPD1), also known as CD39, belongs to the GDA1/CD39 NTPase family. CD39 is primarily expressed on activated lymphoid cells and in endothelial tissues. Kaczmarek [Kaczmarek et al. 1996] demonstrated that CD39, a B-cell activation marker previously characterized by Maliszewski´s group [Maliszewski et al. 1994], encodes vascular ATPDase. It was confirmed to be expressed on the cell surface and to hydrolyze both ATP and ADP equally, and to inhibit platelet aggregation. In the nervous system, it could hydrolyze ATP and other nucleotides to regulate purinergic neurotransmission. Immunohistochemical, Northern, and Western blot analysis showed that CD39 is expressed in epidermal dendritic cells (DC) but not in keratinocyte cell lines. Mizumoto and co-workers [Mizumoto et al. 2002] claimed that CD39 is the dominant Langerhans cell-associated ecto-NTPDase and demonstrated its modulatory roles in inflammation and immune responsiveness. The expression of the CD39 gene was 3.6-fold up-regulated in CD133+ D10 cells, as compared to CD133- D10 cells.

The expression of the **eukaryotic translation elongation factor 1 alpha 2 (EEF1A2)** was 3.6-fold up-regulated in CD133+ D10 cells. EEF1A2 [Lund et al. 1996] encodes an isoform of the alpha subunit of the elongation factor-1 complex, which is responsible for the enzymatic delivery of aminoacyl tRNAs to the ribosome. This isoform (alpha 2) is expressed in brain, heart and skeletal muscle, whereas the other isoform (alpha 1) is expressed in brain, placenta, lung, liver, kidney, and pancreas. Anand and colleagues [Anand et al. 2002] found that the EEF1A2 gene is amplified in 25% of primary ovarian tumours and is highly expressed in approximately 30% of ovarian tumours and established cell lines and thus can be considered a putative oncogene in ovarian cancer [Lee 2003]. They also demonstrated that the EEF1A2 protein has oncogenic properties. Sharma [Sharma et al. 2007] showed that EEF1A2 is highly homologous and functionally similar to the EEF1A1 oncogene, and was found to be restricted only to the normal tissues of the heart, brain, and skeletal muscle. The expression level of EEF1A2 correlates with cell growth but not apoptosis in hepatocellular carcinoma cell lines with different differentiation grades [Grassi et al. 2007] and the overexpression of EEF1A2 and KCIP-1 is associated with lung adenocarcinoma [Li et al. 2006].

Insulin-like growth factor 1 (IGF1) is a member of the large family of insulin-related peptides including insulin, IGF1 and IGF2. The expression of IGF1 was 3-fold up-regulated in CD133+ D10 cells. Insulin-like growth factor binding protein 3 (IGFBP3), the major carrier protein for IGF1 and IGF2, was 2.5fold up-regulated in CD133+ D10 cells. IGF1 mediates many of the growth-promoting effects of growth hormone. Kim [Kim et al. 1991] identified and characterized a promoter regulatory region of the IGF1 gene. Playford´s group [Playford et al. 2000] studied the influence of IGF1 on the interaction between E-cadherin and beta-catenin in human colorectal cancer cells. Their results indicated that IGF1 causes tyrosine phosphorylation and stabilization of beta-catenin. These effects may contribute to transformation, cell migration, and a propensity for increased metastatic potential *in vivo*. IGF1 was reported to be involved in the development of neoplasia. The insulin receptor (IR), insulin-like growth factor receptor (IGFR), and insulin-receptor-related receptor (IRR) form a subgroup of receptor tyrosine kinases that activate the mitogenic MAP kinase signalling cascade. The activated IR regulates cellular uptake and metabolism of fuels, while the activated IGFR promotes cell growth. Hilmi and co-workers [Hilmi et al. 2008] demonstrated that IGF1 promotes resistance to apoptosis in melanoma cells through an increased expression of BCL2, BCL-X(L), and survivin. *In vitro* data from Schlenska-Lange and colleagues [Schlenska-Lange et al.] suggest that IGF1 modulates proliferation and strongly stimulates migration of glioma cell lines. Epidemiological studies demonstrated that high levels of circulating IGF1 might represent a risk factor for different types of cancers, including prostate [Chan et al. 1998], breast [Hankinson et al. 1998], lung [Yu, Berkel 1999; Yu, Rohan 2000] and cervical [Schaffer et al. 2007] tumours. A known cytosine-adenine (CA) repeat polymorphism in the promoter region of the IGF1 gene may affect transcription activity and has been associated with an increased susceptibility to prostate [Chen et al. 2006], breast [Wen et al. 2005] and colorectal cancer [Slattery et al. 2004]. Although results of other studies on this topic [Missmer et al. 2002; DeLellis et al. 2003; Wagner et al. 2004; Cleveland et al. 2006; Figer et al. 2002; Tsuchiya et al. 2005; Li et al. 2004; Friedrichsen et al. 2005; Schildkraut et al. 2005; Nam et al. 2005; Morimoto et al. 2005; Wong et al. 2005] were inconclusive and controversial, Santonocito and co-workers [Santonocito et al. 2008] concluded that an association for IGF1(CA19) and malignant melanoma is in keeping with similar results obtained in prostate or breast cancers, suggesting that this type of repeat may be important in controlling the induction of cancer and its severity. In this study, IGF1 repeats were associated with higher melanoma's Breslow index. However, Chen's group [Chen et al. 2008] showed in a meta-analysis that this (CA)19 repeat polymorphism is unlikely to be a major determinant of susceptibility to cancer on a wide population basis.

The expression of the **CD66** gene, also known as the carcinoembryonic antigen-related cell adhesion molecule 1 (**CEACAM1**, Biliray Glycoprotein 1, BGP), was 3fold up-regulated in CD133+ D10 cells. The carcinoembryonic antigen (CEA) gene family belongs to the immunoglobulin superfamily of genes. The encoded protein was originally described in bile ducts of liver as biliary glycoprotein. Subsequently, it was found to be a cell-cell adhesion molecule detected on leukocytes, epithelia, and endothelia. Multiple cellular activities have been attributed to the specific gene product, including roles in the differentiation and arrangement of tissue three-dimensional structure, angiogenesis, apoptosis, tumor suppression, metastasis, and the modulation of innate and adaptive immune responses. Neumaier [Neumaier et al. 1993] reported that loss or reduced expression of the BGP adhesion molecule is a major event in colorectal carcinogenesis. Ergun and colleagues [Ergün et al. 2000] showed that CEACAM1 exhibits angiogenic properties in *in vitro* and *in vivo* angiogenesis assays. Since CEACAM1 is expressed in tumor microvessels but not in large blood vessels, it may represent a target for the inhibition of tumour angiogenesis. Furthermore, Abou-Rjaily [Abou-Rjaily et al. 2004] reported that CEACAM1 modulates epidermal growth factor receptor-mediated cell proliferation.

The expression of **Proline Dehydrogenase (PRODH) 1**, also known as Proline oxidase 1 (POX) gene, was 2.6 fold up-regulated in CD133+ D10 cells. POX is a p53-induced [Donald et al. 2001] mitochondrial inner-membrane protein that catalyzes the rate-limiting oxidation/dehydrogenation of proline to pyrroline-5-carboxylate (P5C) using cytochrome c and FAD as electron and hydrogen acceptors. In mammals, POX activity is developmentally regulated and tissue specific: highest in liver and kidney, lower in brain and heart and undetectable in most other tissues. It has been shown by Liu's [Liu et al. 2006b] and Maxwell's [Maxwell, Rivera 2003] groups that POX can mediate apoptosis through generation of reactive oxgen species (ROS). Hu and co-workers [Hu et al. 2007] could show that the hyperexpression of POX induces proline-dependent and mitochondria-mediated apoptosis. Rivera et al 2005 proposed that the p53-induces Gene-6 (POX) mediates apoptosis through a calcineurin-dependent pathway. The peroxisome proliferator-activated receptor γ (PPARγ) ligand troglitazone, an anti-diabetic and anti-inflammatory drug, was found to activate the POX promoter and was reported to induce apoptosis, mediated by targeting POX gene expression for generation of ROS by POX both, by PPARγ-dependent and –independent mechanisms. PPARγ ligands have been reported to induce apoptosis in a variety of cancer cells. Proline oxidase, a proapoptotic gene, is induced by troglitazone: evidence for both peroxisome proliferator-activated receptor gamma-dependent (PPARγ) and -independent mechanisms [Pandhare et al. 2006].

TABLE 8   UP-REGULATED GENES IN CD133+ D10 CELLS

FC	GS	APID	Gene Description	ChrLoc
32,4	MGP	202291_s_at	matrix Gla protein	12p13.1-p12.3
27,7	PROM1	204304_s_at	prominin 1	4p15.32
3,8	TPD52	203786_s_at	tumor protein D52-like 1	8q21
3,6	ENTPD1	207691_x_at	ectonucleoside triphosphate diphosphohydrolase 1	10q24
3,6	EEF1A2	204540_at	eukaryotic translation elongation factor 1 alpha 2	20q13.3
3,1	IGF1	209541_at	insulin-like growth factor 1 (somatomedin C)	12q22-q23
3,0	CEACAM1	206576_s_at	carcinoembryonic antigen-related cell adhesion molecule 1 (biliary glycoprotein)	19q13.2
2,7	IGFBP3	210095_s_at	insulin-like growth factor binding protein 3	7p13-p12
2,7	PRODH	214203_s_at	proline dehydrogenase (oxidase) 1	22q11.21
2,4	PDGFC	218718_at	platelet derived growth factor C	4q32
2,1	ADCY2	213217_at	adenylate cyclase 2 (brain)	5p15.3
2,1	UBE2C	202954_at	ubiquitin-conjugating enzyme E2C	20q13.12
2,1	SERPINF1	202283_at	serpin peptidase inhibitor, clade F (alpha-2 antiplasmin, pigment epithelium derived factor), member	17p13.1
2,1	DENND2D	221081_s_at	DENN/MADD domain containing 2D	1p13.3
1,9	CDC2	203213_at	Cell division cycle 2, G1 to S and G2 to M	10q21.1
1,9	HMGCS1	205822_s_at	3-hydroxy-3-methylglutaryl-Coenzyme A synthase 1 (soluble)	5p14-p13
1,9	TMEM16B	220111_s_at	transmembrane protein 16B	12p13.3
1,8	NUP210	213947_s_at	nucleoporin 210kDa	3p25.1
1,8	IFI30	201422_at	interferon, gamma-inducible protein 30	19p13.1
1,8	HJURP	218726_at	Holliday junction recognition protein	2q37.1
1,8	BNIP3	201849_at	BCL2/adenovirus E1B 19kDa interacting protein 3	10q26.3
1,8	LL22NC03-	221901_at	KIAA1644 protein	no data
1,8	MUC7	217059_at	mucin 7, salivary	4q13-q21
1,8	FAM129A	217967_s_at	family with sequence similarity 129, member A	1q25
1,8	CXADR	203917_at	coxsackie virus and adenovirus receptor	21q21.1
1,8	RAB15	59697_at	RAB15, member RAS oncogene family	14q23.3
1,8	HRASLS3	209581_at	HRAS-like suppressor 3	11q12.3-q13.1
1,7	MARCH3	213256_at	membrane-associated ring finger (C3HC4) 3	5q23.2
1,7	ABLIM1	200965_s_at	actin binding LIM protein 1	10q25
1,7	TTC3	210645_s_at	tetratricopeptide repeat domain 3	21q22.2
1,7	SPAG4	219888_at	sperm associated antigen 4	20q11.21
1,7	TCN2	204043_at	transcobalamin II; macrocytic anemia	22q12.2
1,7	RASGRP1	205590_at	RAS guanyl releasing protein 1 (calcium and DAG-regulated)	15q15
1,6	ERG	213541_s_at	v-ets erythroblastosis virus E26 oncogene homolog (avian)	21q22.3
1,6	BTG3	215425_at	BTG family, member 3	21q21.1-q21.2
1,6	KIF23	204709_s_at	kinesin family member 23	15q23
1,6	ADM	202912_at	adrenomedullin	11p15.4
1,6	SLC37A1	218928_s_at	solute carrier family 37 (glycerol-3-phosphate transporter), member 1	21q22.3
1,6	AURKA	208079_s_at	serine/threonine kinase 6 bzw. aurora kinase 6	20q13.2-q13.3
1,5	KIF15	219306_at	kinesin family member 15	3p21.31
1,5	ABHD6	221679_s_at	abhydrolase domain containing 6	3p14.3
1,5	CCNF	204826_at	cyclin F	16p13.3
1,5	SLC22A18AS	206097_at	solute carrier family 22 (organic cation transporter), member 18 antisense	11p15.5
1,5	MICAL2	212473_s_at	microtubule associated monooxygenase, calponin and LIM domain containing 2	11p15.3
1,5	KIF2C	209408_at	kinesin family member 2C	1p34.1
1,5	NRN1	218625_at	neuritin 1	6p25.1
1,5	TM6SF1	219892_at	transmembrane 6 superfamily member 1	15q24-q26
1,5	AMPD3	207992_s_at	adenosine monophosphate deaminase (isoform E)	11p15
1,5	SERGEF	220482_s_at	secretion regulating guanine nucleotide exchange factor	11p14.3
1,4	ZXDC	218639_s_at	ZXD family zinc finger C	3q21.2
1,4	TXNRD3	221906_at	thioredoxin reductase 3	3q21.3
1,4	PSRC1	201896_s_at	proline/serine-rich coiled-coil 1	1p13.3
1,4	ABCA1	203505_at	ATP-binding cassette, sub-family A (ABC1), member 1	9q31.1
1,4	FHOD3	218980_at	formin homology 2 domain containing 3	18q12
1,4	C6orf211	218195_at	chromosome 6 open reading frame 211	6q25.1
1,4	CSRP2	211126_s_at	cysteine and glycine-rich protein 2	12q21.1
1,4	GTSE1	204317_at	G-2 and S-phase expressed 1	22q13.2-q13.3
1,4	BLVRB	202201_at	biliverdin reductase B (flavin reductase (NADPH))	19q13.1-q13.2
1,4	MAFF	36711_at	v-maf musculoaponeurotic fibrosarcoma oncogene homolog F (avian)	22q13.1
1,4	PLS1	205190_at	plastin 1 (I isoform)	3q23
1,4	ALDH9A1	201612_at	aldehyde dehydrogenase 9 family, member A1	1q23.1
1,3	ESPL1	204817_at	extra spindle pole bodies homolog 1 (S. cerevisiae)	12q
1,3	RRH	208314_at	retinal pigment epithelium-derived rhodopsin homolog	4q25
1,3	DCC1	219000_s_at	defective in sister chromatid cohesion homolog 1 (S. cerevisiae)	8q24.12
1,3	LIMS2	220765_s_at	LIM and senescent cell antigen-like domains 2	2q14.2
1,3	ALDOC	202022_at	aldolase C, fructose-bisphosphate	17cen-q12
1,3	HOMER2	217080_s_at	homer homolog 2 (Drosophila)	15q24.3
1,3	DDT	202929_s_at	D-dopachrome tautomerase	22q11.23

Results of gene expression profiling on CD133+ D10 cells. Table shows significantyl (p<0.01) up-regulated genes (>1.3-fold) compared to CD133- D10 cells. **FC** = fold change of up-regulation, **GS** = Gene Symbol, **APID** = Affymetrix Probe ID, **ChrLoc** = chromosomal location.

GENES DOWN-REGULATED MORE THAN 2.5-FOLD (P<0.001) IN CD133+ AS COMPARED TO CD133+ D10 CELLS.

The **tenascin C (TNC)** gene encodes the extracellular cell adhesion molecule TNC, a member of the fibrinogen and fibronectin family. Its expression was more than 4 fold down-regulated in CD133+ compared to the CD133- subpopulation of D10 cells. It belongs to non-structural ECM proteins that are believed to regulate cell adhesion and migration and to have signalling altering functions [Orend, Chiquet-Ehrismann 2000; Hsia, Schwarzbauer 2005]. Tenascin C has been reported to bind integrins, proteoglycans, cell adhesion molecules of the immunoglobulin family and other ECM proteins and to affect both Rho-mediated and Wnt signalling pathways by these complex interactions [Ruiz et al. 2004]. It was also shown to have strong anti-adhesive properties and to counteract cell adhesion to fibronectin by disrupting focal adhesion sites. Tenascin C is expressed in invasive human solid tumours [Sadej et al. 2008]. Tenascin C is involved in extracellular matrix protein-mediated signalling and Neurogenesis, signal transduction, developmental process, ectodermal development and cell communication. Adam and his group [Adám et al. 2006] demonstrated that the tenascin production by fibroblasts in the tumour stroma is directly modulated by melanoma cells mainly through cell-to-cell contact signalling. Tenascin C is heavily involved in cell-cell interactions such resulting in the stimulation of cancerous cell mitogenesis, cell adhesion and antiadhesion. Tenascin C especially inhibits the cell adhesion mediated by fibronectin and may play an important role in the regulation of dynamic changes in ECM.4 [Spring et al. 1989].

Secretogranin II (chromogranin C) was 3.7 fold down-regulated in CD133+ D10 cells. Kirchmair et al. [Kirchmair et al. 1993] reported that secretogranin II belongs to a class of secretory proteins contained in large dense core vesicles of many endocrine cells and neurons. Secretoneurin (SN), a 33-amino acid neuropeptide derived from secretogranin II, is involved in chemotaxis of monocytes and endothelial cells and in regulation of endothelial cell proliferation [Dunzendorfer et al. 1998]. It was demonstrated by Shyu [Shyu et al. 2008] that the expression of SN was markedly upregulated in both, neurons and endothelial cells in a rat model of stroke and in ischemic human brain tissue. Following oxygen and glucose deprivation, SN provided neuroprotection to primary cortical cell cultures. SN also induced expression of the antiapoptotic proteins Bcl2 and Bclxl through the Jak2/Stat3 pathway and inhibited apoptosis by blocking caspase-3 (CASP3) activation. Furthermore, SN injection enhanced stem cell targeting to the injured brain in mice and promoted formation of new blood vessels to increase local cortical blood flow in the ischemic hemisphere. In summary, SN promotes neuroprotection and enhanced neurogenesis and angiogenesis, both in vitro and in vivo.

The gene encoding **STAC** (Src homology 3 and cysteine-rich domains) was 3.5-fold down-regulated in CD133+ D10 cells. According to Suzuki [Suzuki et al. 1996], cysteine-rich and SH3 domains are frequently found in signal transduction proteins and STAC was suggested to be involved in the neuron-specific signal transduction pathway.

The expression of **BCHE** gene encoding butyrylcholinesterase (pseudocholinesterase E1, CHE1, acylcholine acylhydrolase, choline esterase II, cholinesterase), which is located in both the endoplasmatic reticulum and extracellular components, was 3.2-fold down-regulated in CD133+ D10 cells. Various functions of BCHE have been described, including beta-amyloid binding, carboxylesterase activity, cholinesterase activity, enzyme binding and hydrolase activity. Furthermore, it was reported to be involved in the cocaine metabolism, but it has never been associated with the process of melanoma development, formation, metastasis or prognosis. Interestingly, the amino acid sequences of cholinesterase in brain and serum are apparently identical. Cholinesterase is present in particularly high levels in embryonic and foetal human brain as well as in nervous system tumours such as glioblastoma, neuroblastoma, and meningioma. The widespread expression in early differentiation suggests development-related functions for this protein.

As a member of the galectin family, **LGALS1**, a beta-galactoside-binding protein (lectin, galactoside-binding, soluble, 1) was implicated in modulating cell-cell and cell-matrix interactions. LGALS1 (Galectin 1; GAL1) is an endogenous mammalian S-type lectin with highly pleiotropic effect on different tissues. Baldini's group [Baldini et al. 1993] proposed that this gene product may act as an autocrine negative growth factor that regulates cell proliferation in mice with a role in the maintenance of G0 and in the control of cell cycle progression. The expression of Gal-1 was 3.1-fold down-regulated in CD133+ D10. By screening for factors that promote proliferation of mouse neural stem cells in vitro, Sakaguchi and co-workers [Sakaguchi et al. 2006] identified galectin-1. Galectin-1 was found to be expressed in a subset of slowly dividing subventricular zone astrocytes, which included the neural stem cells. Their analysis showed that galectin-1 was an endogenous factor that promoted the proliferation of neural stem cells in adult mouse brain. Data from Kadri et al. [Kadri et al. 2005] suggested that galectin-1 may have a role in immunological functions of human mesenchymal stem cells (MSCs, BMSCs), which were used as a stem cell model in this study. The viability of the lymphoid cells is reduced by gal-1 by triggering apoptosis, however, the mechanism of the gal-1 induced apoptosis is still under investigation. The receptor tyrosine phosphatase, CD45, a heavily glycosylated cell surface molecule binds to gal-1 with high affinity. However, its contribution to the gal-1 induced apoptosis is still controversial [Fajka-Boja et al. 2002; Walzel et al. 1999; Barondes et al. 1994; Perillo et al. 1998; Perillo et al. 1995; Cooper, Barondes 1990; Baum et al. 1995; Pace et al. 2000; Pace et al. 1999]. In melanoma, van den Brûle [van den Brûle et al. 1995] suggested that Galectin-1 modulates cell adhesion to laminin and therefore could be a modulator of invasion and metastasis.

SPOCK encodes a member of a novel Ca(2+)-binding proteoglycan family and its expression was almost 2.8-fold down-regulated in CD133+ D10 cells. Proteoglycans, which consist of a core protein and covalently linked glycosaminoglycans, are components of the extracellular matrix. Bonnet's group [Bonnet et al. 1992] demonstrated that this gene encodes the protein core of a seminal plasma proteoglycan containing chondroitin- and heparan-sulfate chains. The protein's function is unknown, although similarity to thyropin-type cysteine protease-inhibitors suggests its function may be related to protease inhibition. Prenzel et al. [Prenzel et al. 2006] reported a significant overexpression of SPARC/osteonectin mRNA in pancreatic cancer compared to cancer of the papilla of Vater.

TIMP1 (Tissue Inhibitor of MetalloPeptidase 1) belongs to the TIMP gene family. Matrix metalloproteinases (MMPs) are a group of peptidases involved in degradation of the extracellular matrix. The proteins encoded by the TIMP gene family are natural inhibitors of

MMPs and thus prevent ECM degradation. In addition to its inhibitory role against most of the known MMPs, the encoded protein is able to promote cell proliferation in a wide range of cell types, and may also have an anti-apoptotic function. Transcription of this gene is highly inducible in response to many cytokines and hormones. The tissue inhibitor of matrix metalloproteinases-1 (TIMP1) has been recognized as a multifunctional protein. The role of TIMPs in cancer is controversial ranging from an anti-tumour activity to a tumour growth stimulation activity by several mechanisms, including, among others, anti-apoptotic effects [Liu et al. 2003]. In contrast, Ikenaka and co-workers [Ikenaka et al. 2003] recognized that TIMP-1 has a role in inhibiting tumour growth by angiogenesis suppression. The expression of TIMP1 was 2.6-fold down-regulated in CD133+ D10 cells compared to CD133- cell fraction. In a review 2005, Hofmann et al. [Hofmann et al.] summarized the role of matrix metalloproteinases in melanoma cell invasion. Increased expression of TIMPs may have an antimetastatic effect but may also be indicative of a poor prognosis. The latter could be due to growth-stimulating effects of TIMPs on human melanoma cells. On the other hand, TIMPs were shown to inhibit tumour neovascularization. Recent data suggest that this antiangiogenic action of TIMP-2 may rely on matrix metalloproteinase independent mechanisms modulating tumour–host interactions. Interestingly, TIMP1 gene transcription is regulated by RUNX1 and RUNX2 (Cbfa1).

TABLE 9			DOWN-REGULATED GENES IN CD133+ D10 CELLS	
FC	GS	APID	Gene Description	ChrLoc
4,1	TNC	201645_at	tenascin C (hexabrachion)	9q33
3,7	SCG2	204035_at	secretogranin II (chromogranin C)	2q35-q36
3,5	STAC	205743_at	SH3 and cysteine rich domain	3p22.3
3,2	BCHE	205433_at	butyrylcholinesterase	3q26.1-q26.2
3,1	LGALS1	201105_at	lectin, galactoside-binding, soluble, 1 (galectin 1)	22q13.1
2,8	SPOCK1	202363_at	sparc/osteonectin, cwcv and kazal-like domains proteoglycan (testican) 1	5q31
2,6	TIMP1	201666_at	TIMP metallopeptidase inhibitor 1	Xp11.3-p11.23
2,3	FLNA	213746_s_at	filamin A, alpha (actin binding protein 280)	Xq28
2,2	DLK1	209560_s_at	delta-like 1 homolog (Drosophila)	14q32
2,0	SLC7A11	207528_s_at	solute carrier family 7, (cationic amino acid transporter, y+ system) member 11	4q28-q32
1,8	AIM1	212543_at	absent in melanoma 1	6q21
1,8	PTPRD	214043_at	protein tyrosine phosphatase, receptor type, D	9p23-p24.3
1,8	PEG10	212094_at	paternally expressed 10	7q21
1,7	AHNAK	211986_at	AHNAK nucleoprotein	11q12.2
1,6	CBLB	209682_at	Cas-Br-M (murine) ecotropic retroviral transforming sequence b	3q13.11
1,6	BCL2A1	205681_at	BCL2-related protein A1	15q24.3
1,6	CAV1	212097_at	caveolin 1, caveolae protein, 22kDa	7q31.1
1,6	ARMC9	219636_s_at	armadillo repeat containing 9	2q37.1
1,6	SLC27A3	222217_s_at	solute carrier family 27 (fatty acid transporter), member 3	1q21.3
1,6	PLK2	201939_at	polo-like kinase 2 (Drosophila)	5q12.1-q13.2
1,5	EYA2	209692_at	eyes absent homolog 2 (Drosophila)	20q13.1
1,5	LEPREL2	204854_at	leprecan-like 2	12q13
1,5	LSAMP	214460_at	limbic system-associated membrane protein	3q13.2-q21
1,5	JAM3	212813_at	junctional adhesion molecule 3	11q25
1,5	CHI3L2	213060_s_at	chitinase 3-like 2	1p13.3
1,5	QKI	212636_at	quaking homolog, KH domain RNA binding (mouse)	6q26-q27
1,5	EDNRB	204273_at	endothelin receptor type B	13q22
1,4	CITED1	207144_s_at	Cbp/p300-interacting transactivator, with Glu/Asp-rich carboxy-terminal domain, 1	Xq13.1
1,4	WIPF1	202665_s_at	WAS/WASL interacting protein family, member 1	2q31.1
1,4	RAB40B	204547_at	RAB40B, member RAS oncogene family	17q25.3
1,4	RPL17	214291_at	ribosomal protein L17, similar to 60S ribosomal protein L17 (L23)	10q22.1
1,4	SSX1	206626_x_at	synovial sarcoma, X breakpoint 1	Xp11.3-p11.22
1,4	GOLM1	217771_at	golgi membrane protein 1	9q21.33
1,4	SERPINH1	207714_at	serpin peptidase inhibitor, clade H (heat shock protein 47), member 1, (collagen binding protein 1)	11q13.5
1,4	CXCR4	211919_s_at	chemokine (C-X-C motif) receptor 4	2q21
1,4	CINP	217598_at	Cyclin-dependent kinase 2-interacting protein	no data
1,4	SGK1	201739_at	serum/glucocorticoid regulated kinase	6q23
1,4	RAPGEF5	204681_s_at	Rap guanine nucleotide exchange factor (GEF) 5	7p15.3
1,4	RABEPK	203150_at	Rab9 effector protein with kelch motifs	9q33.3
1,4	EIF4E2	213570_at	eukaryotic translation initiation factor 4E family member 2	2q37.1
1,3	SLC1A5	208916_at	solute carrier family 1 (neutral amino acid transporter), member 5	19q13.3
1,3	NOL3	221567_at	nucleolar protein 3 (apoptosis repressor with CARD domain)	16q21-q23
1,3	SLC43A1	204394_at	solute carrier family 43, member 1	11p11.2-p11.1
1,3	KLHL11	220657_at	kelch-like 11 (Drosophila)	17q21.2
1,3	PGBD5	219225_at	piggyBac transposable element derived 5	1q42.13
1,3	FJX1	219522_at	four jointed box 1 (Drosophila)	11p13

Results of gene expression profiling on CD133+ D10 cells. Table shows significantyl (p<0.01) down-regulated genes (>1.3-fold) compared to CD133- D10 cells. **FC** = fold change of up-regulation, **GS** = Gene Symbol, **APID** = Affymetrix Probe ID, **ChrLoc** = chromosomal location.

DISCUSSION

REPETITORIUM
In 1997, Bonnet & Dick [Bonnet, Dick 1997] identified a serially transplantable population of human leukaemia cells enriched for tumour-initiating abilities. By applying a similar experimental protocol to the study of solid tumours, cancer stem cells have now been prospectively identified from human breast and brain cancers, and putative cancer stem cells have been reported in human skin, bone, and prostate tumours, sharing a few properties recently summarized by Ward and Dirks [Ward, Dirks 2007].

CURRENT DEFINITION OF A CANCER STEM CELL
Cancer stem cells should self-renew *in vivo*. Direct evidence of cancer stem cell self-renewal is achieved by observing tumour formation after serially transplanting re-isolated cancer stem cells in secondary and tertiary recipients and by observing re-growth of a phenotypically identical and heterogeneous tumour. Cancer stem cells should demonstrate some differentiation capacity reflecting the tumour from which they were derived. Tumours arising *in vivo* upon injection of isolated putative cancer stem cells should represent a phenocopy of the original tumour. Although there have been speculations that cancer stem cells may originate from transformed stem, progenitor, or differentiated cells, the definition does not imply "per se" any of these origins. For this reason, many investigators prefer the term tumour-initiating cell (TIC).

CURRENT DEFINITION OF A MELANOMA STEM CELL
According to Sabatino's publication [Sabatino et al. 2009] there is recent experimental evidence supporting the existence of a melanoma stem cell phenotype. Fang's group [Fang et al. 2005] described a subset of cells derived from freshly isolated or *in vitro* stabilized melanoma cell lines that was able to form "melanoma spheroids" when grown in a specific stem cell medium. Melanoma stem cells exhibited self-renewal properties after *in vitro* and *in vivo* cloning. The melanoma stem cell-like population exhibited the ability to differentiate into astrocytes or cells of the mesenchymal lineage and was extremely tumourigenic when injected into immune-deficient mice. The spheroids were enriched in CD20 expressing cells. In addition, they expressed CD133 and ABCG2. The expression of these two antigens was

associated with higher tumourigenic potential and ability to create new and bigger spheres [Fang et al. 2005; Monzani et al. 2007].

CHARACTERIZATION OF MELANOMA CELL LINES

This study aimed at investigating whether established melanoma cell lines contain tumour cell subsets that can be referred to as cancer stem cells or tumour-initiating cells. Since CD133+ melanoma cells are rare in clinical samples and difficult to isolate from surgical specimens, the expression of stem cell surface markers, in particular CD133, was analyzed in nine well established human melanoma cell lines, each and every one originally deriving from human metastatic malignant melanomas. The melanoma cell line named WM115 was included in the study because of its previous characterization by Monzani's group in 2007 [Monzani et al. 2007] including a CD133+ phenotype and a strong tumourigenic potential [La Porta et al. 2002].

GENOTYPE

The selection of melanoma cell lines reflects the heterogeneity of the original tumours, and includes highly differentiated cell lines expressing the melanoma differentiation antigens gp100, tyrosinase and MART-1 and undifferentiated cell lines. NANOG, SOX2 and OCT4 genes form a regulatory core essential for maintenance of the undifferentiated state of stem cells and the process of stem cell self-renewal in a complex regulatory network. Hyslop and co-workers [Hyslop et al. 2005] demonstrated that NANOG acts as a gatekeeper of pluripotency in human embryonic stem and carcinoma cells by preventing their differentiation to extraembryonic endoderm and trophectoderm lineages. NANOG expression is high in ES and EC cells and germ cell tumours [Clark et al. 2004] but is down-regulated upon differentiation, concomitant with loss of pluripotency. In the murine system, down-regulation of NANOG expression has been partly attributed to suppression by p53, which was shown to bind to the NANOG promoter region [Lin et al. 2005]. Interestingly, high NANOG expression was detectable on the rather differentiated cell lines D10, WM115 and HBL suggesting that these cell lines either have been misclassified previously or the overexpression of NANOG might also not be obviously linked to the state of differentiation of individual melanoma cell lines.

HOX GENES

The 39 human HOX genes are known for their pivotal role in embryonal development by means of regulating transcription. HOX genes are also known to be expressed in adult differentiated eukaryotic cells, where altered HOX gene in expression uncovered potential functions of HOX genes and their encoded proteins. HOXB7, which was moderately and constantly expressed in all melanoma cell lines investigated, was reported to activate bFGF thereby promoting cellular proliferation in melanomas [Caré et al. 1996]. In the present study there were only marginal differences in HOXB7 expression with a minor down-regulation in HBL cell line. This might suggest a reciprocal correlation of HOXB7 and the apparent state of differentiation in melanoma cell lines. On the other hand, its relatively high and stable mRNA expression levels suggest that HOXB7 may rather be involved in the maintenance of the normal phenotype in melanoma cell lines investigated than in oncogenic transformation [Svingen, Tonissen]. Since HOXC9 and HOXC10 showed similar trends in terms of stability and even higher levels of mRNA expression this could also be applicable to these samples. According to the expression of melanoma differentiation antigens, D10, WM115 and HBL can be considered rather differentiated cell lines. Notably, in our series, only D10, WM115 and HBL expressed HOXC12, suggesting a possible up-regulation of HOXC12 in more differentiated melanoma cell lines.

PHENOTYPE AND CLONOGENIC CAPACITY

Our data indicate that melanoma cell lines do express stem cell surface markers, however their distribution was highly variable. Surprisingly, the expression of CD133 on WM115 cells was not detectable under the conditions used in this study. In contrast with the general thinking that CD133+ cancer stem cells may represent only a very minimal part of the total tumour cell population, CD133 was expressed on high percentages of D10 cells. Furthermore, very small percentages of Me39, RE, Me59 and Na8 cells never exceeding 3% of the total also expressed CD133. CD117 was expressed on virtually all HBL cells indicating that this might represent a specific feature of this highly differentiated cell line. Functional analysis of CD133+ D10 cells demonstrated that the frequency of proliferating CD133+ D10 cells was significantly higher compared to the CD133- fraction. CD105 was the only surface marker investigated that was expressed to different extents on all melanoma cell lines considered in this study but the clonogenic capacity of CD105+ cells was highly variable across samples examined. Furthermore, CD105- cells of Na8 cell line even showed a higher clonogenic capacity compared to the CD105+ fraction. This might suggest that CD105+ expression is not necessarily linked with a higher clonogenic capacity.

GENE EXPRESSION PROFILING

Since CD133 was frequently expressed only on D10 cells, gene expression profiling using Affymetrix® GeneChip® techniques was performed on previously sorted CD133+ and CD133- D10 cells. Genome-wide gene expression profiling of CD133+ D10 cells revealed that only MGP (matrix Gla protein; 32.4-fold) and positive control PROM1 (CD133, prominin1; 27.7-fold), were outstandingly up-regulated across the other 68 up-regulated genes (> 1.3-fold; p=0.001). Further investigations of MGP and PROM1 revealed a more than 50% homology in the promoter sequence of these two genes (data not shown) suggesting a possible transcriptional co-regulation. In addition, IGF and its major corresponding binding protein IGFBP3 were 3.5 and 2.7-fold up-regulated in CD133+ D10 cells, compared to the CD133- fraction. IGF1 plays a key role in the development and growth of multiple tumours and in the prevention of apoptosis. In melanoma cells, IGF1 has been shown to mediate resistance to anoikis-induced apoptosis. Recently, Hilmi and co-workers [Hilmi et al. 2008] could also demonstrated that IGF1 promotes resistance to apoptosis in melanoma cells through an increased expression of BCL2, BCL-X(L), and Survivin. These findings might indicate that the CD133+ phenotype might be associated with resistance to apoptosis in D10 cells thereby supporting its cancer stem cell properties and a higher tumourigenic potential. Inconsistently with findings published by Fang`s group [Fang et al. 2005], CD133+ D10 cells had not up-regulated the expression of ABCG2 which was identified to be over-expressed in primary or metastatic melanoma compared to benign melanocytic nevi [Schatton et al. 2008]. Thus, ABCG2 cannot be considered a marker of melanoma progression in CD133+ D10 cells.

CONCLUSION

Taken together, our data suggest that established melanoma cell lines might represent useful tools for the investigation of functional features of cancer stem cells. Furthermore, gene profiling of CD133+ subset of D10 melanoma cell line has resulted in the identification of one gene, MGP, consistently up-regulated, in comparison with the CD133- subset of the same cell line. Further studies are warranted to validate these results at the gene and protein level, and to assess the potential diagnostic and prognostic relevance of MGP expression in clinical melanoma specimens.

SUMMARY

The characterization of cancer stem cells in tumours of different histological origin represents a goal of high clinical relevance. A major limitation in these studies is represented by the low number of cells endowed with stem properties detectable in clinical specimens. As an alternative it has been proposed that established cell lines might represent useful tools in these studies due to their consistent heterogeneity, even following long term culture. In this work we took advantage of a series of established melanoma cell lines to explore their "stem cell like" characteristics.

Our findings indicate that at least D10 cell line might represent a good model of melanoma stem cells. A D10 subset consistently expressed high levels of CD133. Furthermore, CD133+ D10 cells showed a significantly higher clonogenic capacity than CD133- D10 cells. Most importantly, gene expression profiles of CD133+ and CD133- cells are different, and the expression of at least one gene, encoding matrix Gla protein (MGP), highly significantly correlates with CD133 expression. On the other hand the expression of ABCG2, a proposed marker of melanoma stem cells, was not detectable in CD133+ D10 cells.

Taken together our data suggest that established cell lines could be of use in the analysis of phenotypic and functional features of melanoma stem cell and suggest novel markers of potential clinical relevance.

SUPPLEMENTARY MATERIAL

DETAILED PROTOCOL OF TARGET SYNTHESIS

SYNTHESIS OF COMPLEMENTARY DNA (CDNA)

Total RNA was reverse transcribed with an oligo-dT primer containing a T7 promoter sequence at the 5'-end (T7-Oligo(dT) Promoter Primer, OdT). To prime second strand synthesis, RNA-cDNA hybrids were digested with RNaseH producing patches of single stranded cDNA. The second strand was filled in by DNA polymerase (**FIGURE 6**)

The single reaction components for RNA denaturation and annealing with OdT primer were set up according to the concentration of RNA after RNA Micro-cleanup. The total RNA volume of each condition (samples 1-4) containing $5\mu g$ RNA was incubated with $2.5\mu l$ of a mix comprised of a previously in H_2O diluted Poly-A RNA control solution (1:3.5) and the OdT mix. The reactions were set up in 0.5ml tubes on ice. The total reaction volume of $12\ \mu l$ per tube was achieved by adjusting missing volumes with H_2O. After full-speed-vortexing for 2s and pulse-spinning, the tubes were placed in the thermal cycler at 70°C for exactly 10min. Afterwards, samples were put on ice for 3min and the thermal cycler was set up waiting at 42°C. The samples were then centrifuged full speed (14.000rpm) for 20s and placed back on ice. The 1st Strand Master Mix was prepared on ice comprising 5x concentrated 1st Strand Buffer, DTT and dNTP and $7\mu l$ of the 1st Strand Master Mix was applied to each sample. The tubes were placed in the thermal cycler for 2min at 42°C and the samples were incubated with $1\mu l$ reverse transcriptase (SuperScript RT II) up to a total volume of $20\mu l$ per tube. Following the incubation at 42°C for 1h, the samples were replaced on ice. The preparation of the 2nd Strand Master Mix was carried out using 5x concentrated 2nd Strand Buffer, 10mM dNTP and H_2O. The mix was vortexed briefly before adding the 2nd strand enzymes, including $10U/\mu l$ *E.coli* DNA Ligase, $10U/\mu l$ *E.coli* DNA Polymerase I and $2U/\mu l$ *E.coli* RNase H. Each sample obtained $130\mu l$ 2nd Strand Master Mix up to a total reaction volume of $150\mu l$. The tubes were placed in the thermal cycler at 16°C for 2h. After these 2h of incubation, each reaction mix was incubated with $2\mu l$ T4 DNA Polymerase for further 5min. Following Rnase H-mediated second strand cDNA synthesis, the double stranded cDNA needed to be purified and served as a template for the subsequent *in vitro* transcription (IVT). Before proceeding to cDNA cleanup, $10\mu l$ of 0.5M EDTA were added to each sample. In order to purify cDNA, the total reaction volume of now $162\mu l$ was transferred into 1.5ml tubes, preloaded with $600\mu l$

cDNA Binding Buffer. Following vortexing and pulse-spinning, 500µl of the sample (762 µl) were applied onto cDNA Cleanup Spin Columns and centrifuged at 12.000rpm for 1min. The flow-through was discarded and the spin column was reloaded with the remaining volume of the sample (262µl). After the flow-through was again discarded, the spin column was transferred onto new 2ml collection tubes. 750µl of the cDNA Wash Buffer were applied onto the spin column, centrifuged at 12.000rpm for 1min and the flow-through was discarded afresh. The spin columns were centrifuged again but this time lid-opened at 14.000rpm for 5min. Both, the flow-through and collection tubes were discarded and the spin column was transferred onto new 1.5ml tubes. Subsequently, 23µl of cDNA Elution Buffer were applied directly onto the middle of the spin column membrane without touching it and the reaction was incubated at room temperature for 1min. The samples were placed in the centrifuge at 14.000rpm for 1min to elute. The eluate was vortexed and pulse-spun. Exactly 20µl of the eluate had to be transferred into new 0.5ml tubes to proceed to the transcription of cDNA into cRNA (IVT).

SYNTHESIS OF BIOTIN-LABELLED ANTISENSE CRNA
Review FIGURE 6. The double stranded cDNA served as a template for T7 RNA polymerase-driven *in vitro* transcription (IVT) which yielded up to 100X the starting mRNA pool. At room temperature, 20µl of the IVT Master Mix, containing 10x concentrated IVT Labelling Buffer, IVT Labelling NTP Mix and IVT Labelling Enzyme Mix, were assembled with 20µl of purified cDNA by pipetting and pulse-spinning. The IVT reaction was carried out in a thermal cycler at 37°C for 16h. RNA probes were labelled in the second round of IVT with biotinylated nucleotides (ENZO, Farmingdale, NY). Overall amplification was estimated to be ≥10.000 fold (Gallardo et al. 2003). The overnight-synthesized biotin-labelled antisense cRNA (IVT) needed to be purified the next day using cRNA Sample Cleanup Module (Affymetrix, UK). In order to reach 100µl total volume, 60µl RNAse-free water was applied to each IVT reaction. The entire volume was then transferred in new 1.5ml tubes, preloaded with 350µl cRNA Binding Buffer, vortexed and pulse-spun. The reaction volume was filled up with 250µl absolute ethanol to a final volume of 700µl. The mixture was applied onto IVT cRNA Cleanup Spin Columns placed on 2ml tubes and centrifuged at 12.000rpm for 20s. Following centrifugation, flow-through and collection tubes were discarded and the spin

columns were transferred to new 2ml collection tubes in order to be washed with 500µl of IVT cRNA Wash Buffer at 12.000rpm for 20s. The flow-through was discarded, 500µl of 80% ethanol were applied onto the spin column and the samples were centrifuged again at 12.000rpm for 20s. Following centrifugation, the flow-through was discarded and the samples were centrifuged lid-opened again at 14.000rpm for 5min. Both, flow-through and collection tubes were discarded and the spin columns were transferred on new 1.5ml low-binding in order to be loaded with 26µl RNAse-free water. The tubes were placed in the centrifuge for 1min at 14.000rpm to elute. The eluate was vortex and puls-spun and the purified cRNA was incubated on ice. To assess the amount of target (cRNA) produced and purified, the absorbance and the 260/280 ratio was assessed using a spectrophotometer (NanoDrop). Expected values ranged from 1000 to 3000ng/µl. Aliquots of the IVT products of 1µl were mixed with 2µl H$_2$O and gel electrophoresis was done on these samples in order to estimate the yield and size distribution of labelled transcripts. FIGURE 8 shows the results of unfragmented cRNA products examined on an Agilent 2100 Bioanalyzer.

FRAGMENTATION OF BIOTIN-LABELLED ANTISENSE CRNA

Following cRNA cleanup and quantification, biotin-labelled antisense cRNA (target) was fragmented before hybridization onto GeneChip® probe arrays, using 5x concentrated Fragmentation Buffer, designed to break down full-length cRNA to 35 to 200 base fragments by metal-induced hydrolysis. The 35µl of fragmentation reaction composed of 7µl 5x concentrated Fragmentation Buffer, the appropriate volume for 17.5µg cRNA and variable amounts of RNase-free water. Following 35min of incubation at 94°C in a thermal cycler, samples were put on ice and an aliquot of each sample was saved for fragment analysis on the Bioanalyzer. FIGURE 8 shows the results of fragmented cRNA products examined on an Agilent 2100 Bioanalyzer. Undiluted, fragmented sample RNA was stored at -70°C until ready to perform hybridization.

HYBRIDIZATION ONTO AFFYMETRIX GENECHIP®

Hybridization Cocktail Master Mix was set up on ice comprising of 2x concentrated Hybridization Mix, Control Oligonucleotide B2 (3nM), 20x concentrated Eukaryotic Hybridization Controls, DMSO and H$_2$O. The Master Mix was mixed by vortexing and 180µl were distributed into new series of 0.5ml tubes. For the hybridization of each sample, 20µl of fragmented cRNA were provided and applied onto the Master Mix. Gene chips and 1x concentrated Hybridization Buffer, stored at 4°C, were equilibrated to room temperature 5 to 10min before use. The Hybridization oven was set up to 45°C and the targets (cRNA in Hybridization cocktail) were thawed, pulse-spun and denaturised in a thermal cycler for 5min at 99°C before going to 45°C for further 5min. Immediately after the denaturation of the targets was induced, and gene chips were filled with 200µl of Pre-Hybridization Mix and incubated at 45°C for 10min in the hybridization oven with rotation at 60rpm. The hybridization cocktail was centrifuged at maximum speed for 5 min to collect any insoluble material from the hybridization mixture. The probe arrays were removed from the hybridization oven and the arrays were vent with a clean pipette tip and the Pre-Hybridization Mix was extracted. Finally, the probe arrays were refilled with the appropriate volume of the clarified hybridization cocktail and placed for exactly 16h into the hybridization oven, set to 45°C and rotating at 60rpm. During the latter part of the 16h-hybridization the reagents for the washing and staining steps, required immediately after completion of hybridization, were prepared. For an overview review again **FIGURE 6** and **FIGURE 9**.

WASHING, STAINING AND SCANNING PROBE ARRAYS

The 11µm feature size arrays were washed and stained on a Fluidics Station 450 (Affymetrix) by using the Hybridization Wash and Stain Kit (Affymetrix, Cat# 900720). In order to increase the signal strength, the antibody amplification protocol FS450_0002 was used (http://www.affymetrix.com). This protocol required two different types of washing buffer, a staining buffer and two distinguishing staining solutions. All solutions were prepared during the latter part of hybridization. In order to prepare 1000ml non-stringent Wash Buffer A (6X SSPE, 0.01% Tween-20), 300 ml of 20X SSPE, 1.0ml of 10% Tween-20 and 699ml H_2O were mixed and filtered through a 0.2µm filter. Stringent Wash Buffer B (100 mM MES, 0.1M [Na+], 0.01% Tween-20) was prepared using 83.3ml of 12x concentrated MES Stock Buffer, 5.2ml of 5 M NaCl, 1.0ml of 10% Tween-20 and 910.5ml H_2O for a total volume of 1000ml. Wash Buffer B was also filter through a 0.2µm filter and both types of washing buffer were store at 2°C to 8°C, shielded from light. 250 ml of 2x concentrated Stain Buffer (Final 1X concentration: 100mM MES, 1 M [Na+], 0.05% Tween-20) were prepared using

41.7ml of 12x concentrated MES Stock Buffer, 92.5ml of 5 M NaCl, 2.5ml of 10% Tween-20 and 113.3ml H_2O were mixed, filtered through a 0.2μm filter and stored at 2°C to 8°C, shield from light. The Fluidics Station 450, operated using Affymetrix® Microarray Suite or GeneChip® Operating Software (GCOS), was used to wash and stain the probe arrays. After 16h of hybridization, the hybridization cocktail was removed from the probe array and it was completely refilled with the appropriate volume of Non-Stringent Wash Buffer (Wash Buffer A). Probe arrays were stored at 4°C before proceeding with washing and staining. Probe arrays were stained with two different types of staining reagents, including Streptavidin Phycoerythrin (SAPE) Stain Solution and Antibody Solution Mix. SAPE Stain Solution Mix was prepared using 600μl 2x concentrated Stain Buffer, 48.0μl BSA (50mg/ml), 12μl SAPE (1mg/ml Streptavidin Phycoerythrin) and 540.0μl de-ionized (DI-) H_2O. The solution was mixed and divided into two aliquots of 600μl each to be used for the 1st and 2nd stain of the Fluidics Protocol, which is described in the next stanza. The Antibody Solution Mix comprised of 300μl 2x concentrated Stain Buffer, 24.0μl BSA (50mg/ml), 6μl Goat IgG Stock (10mg/ml), 3.6μl biotinylated antibody (0.5mg/ml) and 266.4μl DI-H_2O up to a total volume of 600μl. Antibody Solution Mix was used for the 3rd stain of the Fluidics Protocol.

ANTIBODY AMPLIFICATION FOR EUKARYOTIC TARGETS
Sample holders of the fluidics station were loaded with micro centrifuge vials preloaded with the required staining solutions at which 600μl of the vial filled with SAPE Staining Solution were put in the sample holders 1 and 3 and 600μl of the vial containing the Antibody Staining Solution was placed in sample holder 2. The needle lever was pressed down in order to snap needles into position and to start the run. At the end of the run, micro centrifuge vials were removed from the sample holders and replaced with three empty micro centrifuge vials. The probe arrays were also removed from the fluidics station and the probe array window was checked for optionally present bubbles or air pockets which would have to be removed. If the probe array had no large bubbles it was ready for scanning with GeneChip® Scanner 3000 controlled by Affymetrix® GeneChip® Operating System (GCOS). For the Fluidics Protocol FS450_002 see http://www.affymetrix.com.

STATISTICAL ANALYSIS OF EXPRESSION DATA

In the GeneChip® system a known gene or potentially expressed sequence is represented on the chip by 11-20 unique oligomeric probes, each 25 bases in length. The group of probes corresponding to a given gene or small group of highly similar genes is known as the probe set and generally spans a region of about 600 bases, known as the target sequence. Many copies of each oligomer are synthesized in discrete features (or cells) on the GeneChip® array. In addition, for each oligomer on the array there is a matched oligomer, synthesized in an adjacent cell that is identical with the exception of a mismatched base at the central position (i.e. base 13). These are designated Perfect Match (PM) and Mismatch (MM) probes, respectively (**FIGURE 9**). Probes that are complementary to the sequence of interest are called perfect match (PM), probes that are complementary to the sequence of interest except for homomeric base change (A-T or G-C) at the 13th position are called mismatch (MM). The MM probes serves as a control for non-specific hybridization. In order to obtain gene expression measured probe intensities needed to be combined. Using GCOS, the Affymetrix program generated raw data (not normalized). Within GeneSpring® raw data were preprocessed including background adjustment, normalization, and summarization of probe sets, using the GeneChip® Robust Multiarray Analysis (GC-RMA). Genes whose signals were lower than background in all gene chips were filtered out, subsequently genes were filtered based on fold change. Statistical analysis on the gene expression profile were performed by using Fisher`s analysis of variance (ANOVA).

REFERENCES

Abou-Rjaily, George A.; Lee, Sang Jun; May, Denisa; Al-Share, Qusai Y.; Deangelis, Anthony M.; Ruch, Randall J. et al. (2004): CEACAM1 modulates epidermal growth factor receptor--mediated cell proliferation. In: The Journal of clinical investigation, Jg. 114, H. 7, S. 944–952.

Adám, Balázs; Tóth, László; Pásti, Gabriella; Balázs, Margit; Adány, Róza (2006): Contact stimulation of fibroblasts for tenascin production by melanoma cells. In: Melanoma research, Jg. 16, H. 5, S. 385–391.

Al-Hajj, Muhammad; Wicha, Max S.; Benito-Hernandez, Adalberto; Morrison, Sean J.; Clarke, Michael F. (2003): Prospective identification of tumorigenic breast cancer cells. In: Proceedings of the National Academy of Sciences of the United States of America, Jg. 100, H. 7, S. 3983–3988.

Anand, Nisha; Murthy, Sabita; Amann, Gudrun; Wernick, Meredith; Porter, Lisa A.; Cukier, I. Howard et al. (2002): Protein elongation factor EEF1A2 is a putative oncogene in ovarian cancer. In: Nature genetics, Jg. 31, H. 3, S. 301–305.

Austin, T. W.; Solar, G. P.; Ziegler, F. C.; Liem, L.; Matthews, W. (1997): A role for the Wnt gene family in hematopoiesis: expansion of multilineage progenitor cells. In: Blood, Jg. 89, H. 10, S. 3624–3635.

Baldini, A.; Gress, T.; Patel, K.; Muresu, R.; Chiariotti, L.; Williamson, P. et al. (1993): Mapping on human and mouse chromosomes of the gene for the beta-galactoside-binding protein, an autocrine-negative growth factor. In: Genomics, Jg. 15, H. 1, S. 216–218.

Bao, Shideng; Wu, Qiulian; McLendon, Roger E.; Hao, Yueling; Shi, Qing; Hjelmeland, Anita B. et al. (2006): Glioma stem cells promote radioresistance by preferential activation of the DNA damage response. In: Nature, Jg. 444, H. 7120, S. 756–760.

Barondes, S. H.; Castronovo, V.; Cooper, D. N.; Cummings, R. D.; Drickamer, K.; Feizi, T. et al. (1994): Galectins: a family of animal beta-galactoside-binding lectins. In: Cell, Jg. 76, H. 4, S. 597–598.

Baum, L. G.; Seilhamer, J. J.; Pang, M.; Levine, W. B.; Beynon, D.; Berliner, J. A. (1995): Synthesis of an endogeneous lectin, galectin-1, by human endothelial cells is up-regulated by endothelial cell activation. In: Glycoconjugate journal, Jg. 12, H. 1, S. 63–68.

Bidlingmaier, Scott; Zhu, Xiaodong; Liu, Bin (2008): The utility and limitations of glycosylated human CD133 epitopes in defining cancer stem cells. In: Journal of molecular medicine (Berlin, Germany), Jg. 86, H. 9, S. 1025–1032.

Bonnet, D.; Dick, J. E. (1997): Human acute myeloid leukemia is organized as a hierarchy that originates from a primitive hematopoietic cell. In: Nature medicine, Jg. 3, H. 7, S. 730–737.

Bonnet, F.; Perin, J. P.; Maillet, P.; Jolles, P.; Alliel, P. M. (1992): Characterization of a human seminal plasma glycosaminoglycan-bearing polypeptide. In: The Biochemical journal, Jg. 288 (Pt 2), S. 565–569.

Boutros, Rose; Fanayan, Susan; Shehata, Mona; Byrne, Jennifer A. (2004): The tumor protein D52 family: many pieces, many puzzles. In: Biochemical and biophysical research communications, Jg. 325, H. 4, S. 1115–1121.

Byrne, J. A.; Mattei, M. G.; Basset, P. (1996): Definition of the tumor protein D52 (TPD52) gene family through cloning of D52 homologues in human (hD53) and mouse (mD52). In: Genomics, Jg. 35, H. 3, S. 523–532.

Calvo, R.; Drabkin, H. A. (2000): Embryonic genes in cancer. In: Annals of oncology : official journal of the European Society for Medical Oncology / ESMO, Jg. 11 Suppl 3, S. 207–218.

Cancela, L.; Hsieh, C. L.; Francke, U.; Price, P. A. (1990): Molecular structure, chromosome assignment, and promoter organization of the human matrix Gla protein gene. In: The Journal of biological chemistry, Jg. 265, H. 25, S. 15040–15048.

Cantile, M.; Pettinato, G.; Procino, A.; Feliciello, I.; Cindolo, L.; Cillo, C. (2003): In vivo expression of the whole HOX gene network in human breast cancer. In: European journal of cancer (Oxford, England : 1990), Jg. 39, H. 2, S. 257–264.

Caré, A.; Silvani, A.; Meccia, E.; Mattia, G.; Stoppacciaro, A.; Parmiani, G. et al. (1996): HOXB7 constitutively activates basic fibroblast growth factor in melanomas. In: Molecular and cellular biology, Jg. 16, H. 9, S. 4842–4851.

Carè, A.; Felicetti, F.; Meccia, E.; Bottero, L.; Parenza, M.; Stoppacciaro, A. et al. (2001): HOXB7: a key factor for tumor-associated angiogenic switch. In: Cancer research, Jg. 61, H. 17, S. 6532–6539.

Carmeliet, P.; Jain, R. K. (2000): Angiogenesis in cancer and other diseases. In: Nature, Jg. 407, H. 6801, S. 249–257.

Chan, E. F.; Gat, U.; McNiff, J. M.; Fuchs, E. (1999): A common human skin tumour is caused by activating mutations in beta-catenin. In: Nature genetics, Jg. 21, H. 4, S. 410–413.

Chan, J. M.; Stampfer, M. J.; Giovannucci, E.; Gann, P. H.; Ma, J.; Wilkinson, P. et al. (1998): Plasma insulin-like growth factor-I and prostate cancer risk: a prospective study. In: Science (New York, N.Y.), Jg. 279, H. 5350, S. 563–566.

Chang, Howard Y.; Chi, Jen-Tsan; Dudoit, Sandrine; Bondre, Chanda; van de Rijn, Matt; Botstein, David; Brown, Patrick O. (2002): Diversity, topographic differentiation, and positional memory in human fibroblasts. In: Proceedings of the National Academy of Sciences of the United States of America, Jg. 99, H. 20, S. 12877–12882.

Chen, Chu; Freeman, Robert; Voigt, Lynda F.; Fitzpatrick, Annette; Plymate, Stephen R.; Weiss, Noel S. (2006): Prostate cancer risk in relation to selected genetic polymorphisms in insulin-like growth factor-I, insulin-like growth factor binding protein-3, and insulin-like growth factor-I receptor. In: Cancer epidemiology, biomarkers & prevention : a publication of the American Association for Cancer Research, cosponsored by the American Society of Preventive Oncology, Jg. 15, H. 12, S. 2461–2466.

Chen, L.; O'Bryan, J. P.; Smith, H. S.; Liu, E. (1990): Overexpression of matrix Gla protein mRNA in malignant human breast cells: isolation by differential cDNA hybridization. In: Oncogene, Jg. 5, H. 9, S. 1391–1395.

Chen, Xin; Guan, Jianming; Song, Yuting; Chen, Peilin; Zheng, Hongxia; Tang, Cheng; Wu, Qihan (2008): IGF-I (CA) repeat polymorphisms and risk of cancer: a meta-analysis. In: Journal of human genetics, Jg. 53, H. 3, S. 227–238.

Cheng, Chien-Jui; Wu, Yu-Chih; Shu, Jye-An; Ling, Thai-Yen; Kuo, Hung-Chih; Wu, Jui-Yu et al. (2007a): Aberrant expression and distribution of the OCT-4 transcription factor in seminomas. In: Journal of biomedical science, Jg. 14, H. 6, S. 797–807.

Cheng, L.; Sung, M-T; Cossu-Rocca, P.; Jones, T. D.; MacLennan, G. T.; Jong, J. de et al. (2007b): OCT4: biological functions and clinical applications as a marker of germ cell neoplasia. In: The Journal of pathology, Jg. 211, H. 1, S. 1–9.

Chung, Eun Joo; Hwang, Sang-Gu; Nguyen, PhuongMai; Lee, Sunmin; Kim, Jung-Sik; Kim, Jin Woo et al. (2002): Regulation of leukemic cell adhesion, proliferation, and survival by beta-catenin. In: Blood, Jg. 100, H. 3, S. 982–990.

Cillo, C.; Barba, P.; Freschi, G.; Bucciarelli, G.; Magli, M. C.; Boncinelli, E. (1992): HOX gene expression in normal and neoplastic human kidney. In: International journal of cancer. Journal international du cancer, Jg. 51, H. 6, S. 892–897.

Cillo, C.; Faiella, A.; Cantile, M.; Boncinelli, E. (1999): Homeobox genes and cancer. In: Experimental cell research, Jg. 248, H. 1, S. 1–9.

Clark, Amander T.; Rodriguez, Ryan T.; Bodnar, Megan S.; Abeyta, Michael J.; Cedars, Marcelle I.; Turek, Paul J. et al. (2004): Human STELLAR, NANOG, and GDF3 genes are expressed in pluripotent cells and map to chromosome 12p13, a hotspot for teratocarcinoma. In: Stem cells (Dayton, Ohio), Jg. 22, H. 2, S. 169–179.

Cleveland, Rebecca J.; Gammon, Marilie D.; Edmiston, Sharon N.; Teitelbaum, Susan L.; Britton, Julie A.; Terry, Mary Beth et al. (2006): IGF1 CA repeat polymorphisms, lifestyle factors and breast cancer risk in the Long Island Breast Cancer Study Project. In: Carcinogenesis, Jg. 27, H. 4, S. 758–765.

Collins, Anne T.; Berry, Paul A.; Hyde, Catherine; Stower, Michael J.; Maitland, Norman J. (2005): Prospective identification of tumorigenic prostate cancer stem cells. In: Cancer research, Jg. 65, H. 23, S. 10946–10951.

Cooper, D. N.; Barondes, S. H. (1990): Evidence for export of a muscle lectin from cytosol to extracellular matrix and for a novel secretory mechanism. In: The Journal of cell biology, Jg. 110, H. 5, S. 1681–1691.

DeLellis, K.; Ingles, S.; Kolonel, L.; McKean-Cowdin, R.; Henderson, B.; Stanczyk, F.; Probst-Hensch, N. M. (2003): IGF1 genotype, mean plasma level and breast cancer risk in the Hawaii/Los Angeles multiethnic cohort. In: British journal of cancer, Jg. 88, H. 2, S. 277–282.

Dellatore, Shara M.; Garcia, A. Sofia; Miller, William M. (2008): Mimicking stem cell niches to increase stem cell expansion. In: Current opinion in biotechnology, Jg. 19, H. 5, S. 534–540.

Donald, S. P.; Sun, X. Y.; Hu, C. A.; Yu, J.; Mei, J. M.; Valle, D.; Phang, J. M. (2001): Proline oxidase, encoded by p53-induced gene-6, catalyzes the generation of proline-dependent reactive oxygen species. In: Cancer research, Jg. 61, H. 5, S. 1810–1815.

Dunzendorfer, S.; Schratzberger, P.; Reinisch, N.; Kähler, C. M.; Wiedermann, C. J. (1998): Secretoneurin, a novel neuropeptide, is a potent chemoattractant for human eosinophils. In: Blood, Jg. 91, H. 5, S. 1527–1532.

Ergün, S.; Kilik, N.; Ziegeler, G.; Hansen, A.; Nollau, P.; Götze, J. et al. (2000): CEA-related cell adhesion molecule 1: a potent angiogenic factor and a major effector of vascular endothelial growth factor. In: Molecular cell, Jg. 5, H. 2, S. 311–320.

Fajka-Boja, Roberta; Szemes, Marianna; Ion, Gabriela; Légrádi, Adám; Caron, Michel; Monostori, Eva (2002): Receptor tyrosine phosphatase, CD45 binds galectin-1 but does not mediate its apoptotic signal in T cell lines. In: Immunology letters, Jg. 82, H. 1-2, S. 149–154.

Fang, Dong; Nguyen, Thiennga K.; Leishear, Kim; Finko, Rena; Kulp, Angela N.; Hotz, Susan et al. (2005): A tumorigenic subpopulation with stem cell properties in melanomas. In: Cancer research, Jg. 65, H. 20, S. 9328–9337.

Favier, B.; Dollé, P. (1997): Developmental functions of mammalian Hox genes. In: Molecular human reproduction, Jg. 3, H. 2, S. 115–131.

Fearon, E. R.; Burke, P. J.; Schiffer, C. A.; Zehnbauer, B. A.; Vogelstein, B. (1986a): Differentiation of leukemia cells to polymorphonuclear leukocytes in patients with acute nonlymphocytic leukemia. In: The New England journal of medicine, Jg. 315, H. 1, S. 15–24.

Fearon, E. R.; Burke, P. J.; Zehnbauer, B. A.; Vogelstein, B.; Schiffer, C. A. (1986b): Differentiation of blast cells in acute nonlymphocytic leukemia. In: The New England journal of medicine, Jg. 315, H. 23, S. 1488.

Figer, Arie; Karasik, Yael Patael; Baruch, Ruth Gershoni; Chetrit, Angela; Papa, Moshe Z.; Sade, Revital Bruchim Bar et al. (2002): Insulin-like growth factor I polymorphism and breast cancer risk in Jewish women. In: The Israel Medical Association journal : IMAJ, Jg. 4, H. 10, S. 759–762.

Fong, Helen; Hohenstein, Kristi A.; Donovan, Peter J. (2008): Regulation of self-renewal and pluripotency by Sox2 in human embryonic stem cells. In: Stem cells (Dayton, Ohio), Jg. 26, H. 8, S. 1931–1938.

Frank, Natasha Y.; Margaryan, Armen; Huang, Ying; Schatton, Tobias; Waaga-Gasser, Ana Maria; Gasser, Martin et al. (2005): ABCB5-mediated doxorubicin transport and chemoresistance in human malignant melanoma. In: Cancer research, Jg. 65, H. 10, S. 4320–4333.

Friedrichsen, Danielle M.; Hawley, Sarah; Shu, Jainfen; Humphrey, Mariela; Sabacan, Leah; Iwasaki, Lori et al. (2005): IGF-I and IGFBP-3 polymorphisms and risk of prostate cancer. In: The Prostate, Jg. 65, H. 1, S. 44–51.

Frisan, T.; Levitsky, V.; Masucci, M. (2001): Limiting dilution assay. In: Methods in molecular biology (Clifton, N.J.), Jg. 174, S. 213–216.

Garbe, Claus; Hauschild, Axel; Volkenandt, Matthias; Schadendorf, Dirk; Stolz, Wilhelm; Reinhold, Uwe et al. (2008a): Evidence-based and interdisciplinary consensus-based German guidelines: systemic medical treatment of melanoma in the adjuvant and palliative setting. In: Melanoma research, Jg. 18, H. 2, S. 152–160.

Garbe, Claus; Hauschild, Axel; Volkenandt, Matthias; Schadendorf, Dirk; Stolz, Wilhelm; Reinhold, Uwe et al. (2008b): Evidence and interdisciplinary consensus-based German guidelines: surgical treatment and radiotherapy of melanoma. In: Melanoma research, Jg. 18, H. 1, S. 61–67.

Garbe, Claus; Schadendorf, Dirk; Stolz, Wilhelm; Volkenandt, Matthias; Reinhold, Uwe; Kortmann, Rolf-Dieter et al. (2008c): Short German guidelines: malignant melanoma. In: Journal der Deutschen Dermatologischen Gesellschaft = Journal of the German Society of Dermatology : JDDG, Jg. 6 Suppl 1, S. S9-S14.

Gat, U.; DasGupta, R.; Degenstein, L.; Fuchs, E. (1998): De Novo hair follicle morphogenesis and hair tumors in mice expressing a truncated beta-catenin in skin. In: Cell, Jg. 95, H. 5, S. 605–614.

Gheduzzi, Dealba; Boraldi, Federica; Annovi, Giulia; DeVincenzi, Chiara Paolinelli; Schurgers, Leon J.; Vermeer, Cees et al. (2007): Matrix Gla protein is involved in elastic fiber calcification in the dermis of pseudoxanthoma elasticum patients. In: Laboratory investigation; a journal of technical methods and pathology, Jg. 87, H. 10, S. 998–1008.

Grassi, G.; Scaggiante, B.; Farra, R.; Dapas, B.; Agostini, F.; Baiz, D. et al. (2007): The expression levels of the translational factors eEF1A 1/2 correlate with cell growth but not apoptosis in hepatocellular carcinoma cell lines with different differentiation grade. In: Biochimie, Jg. 89, H. 12, S. 1544–1552.

Gruss, P.; Kessel, M. (1991): Axial specification in higher vertebrates. In: Current opinion in genetics & development, Jg. 1, H. 2, S. 204–210.

Hale, J. E.; Williamson, M. K.; Price, P. A. (1991): Carboxyl-terminal proteolytic processing of matrix Gla protein. In: The Journal of biological chemistry, Jg. 266, H. 31, S. 21145–21149.

Hamburger, A.; Salmon, S. E. (1977): Primary bioassay of human myeloma stem cells. In: The Journal of clinical investigation, Jg. 60, H. 4, S. 846–854.

Hankinson, S. E.; Willett, W. C.; Colditz, G. A.; Hunter, D. J.; Michaud, D. S.; Deroo, B. et al. (1998): Circulating concentrations of insulin-like growth factor-I and risk of breast cancer. In: Lancet, Jg. 351, H. 9113, S. 1393–1396.

Hart, Adam H.; Hartley, Lynne; Ibrahim, Marilyn; Robb, Lorraine (2004): Identification, cloning and expression analysis of the pluripotency promoting Nanog genes in mouse and human. In: Developmental dynamics : an official publication of the American Association of Anatomists, Jg. 230, H. 1, S. 187–198.

Hendig, Doris; Zarbock, Ralf; Szliska, Christiane; Kleesiek, Knut; Götting, Christian (2008): The local calcification inhibitor matrix Gla protein in pseudoxanthoma elasticum. In: Clinical biochemistry, Jg. 41, H. 6, S. 407–412.

Hermans, Marc M. H.; Vermeer, Cees; Kooman, Jeroen P.; Brandenburg, Vincent; Ketteler, Markus; Gladziwa, Ulrich et al. (2007): Undercarboxylated matrix GLA protein levels are decreased in dialysis patients and related to parameters of calcium-phosphate metabolism and aortic augmentation index. In: Blood purification, Jg. 25, H. 5-6, S. 395–401.

Hilmi, Caroline; Larribere, Lionel; Giuliano, Sandy; Bille, Karine; Ortonne, Jean-Paul; Ballotti, Robert; Bertolotto, Corine (2008): IGF1 promotes resistance to apoptosis in melanoma cells through an increased expression of BCL2, BCL-X(L), and survivin. In: The Journal of investigative dermatology, Jg. 128, H. 6, S. 1499–1505.

Hofmann, Uta B.; Houben, Roland; Bröcker, Eva-B; Becker, Jürgen C.: Role of matrix metalloproteinases in melanoma cell invasion. In: Biochimie, Jg. 87, H. 3-4, S. 307–314.

Hsia, Henry C.; Schwarzbauer, Jean E. (2005): Meet the tenascins: multifunctional and mysterious. In: The Journal of biological chemistry, Jg. 280, H. 29, S. 26641–26644.

Hu, Chien-an A.; Donald, Steven P.; Yu, Jian; Lin, Wei-Wen; Liu, Zhihe; Steel, Gary et al. (2007): Overexpression of proline oxidase induces proline-dependent and mitochondria-mediated apoptosis. In: Molecular and cellular biochemistry, Jg. 295, H. 1-2, S. 85–92.

Hyslop, Louise; Stojkovic, Miodrag; Armstrong, Lyle; Walter, Theresia; Stojkovic, Petra; Przyborski, Stefan et al. (2005): Downregulation of NANOG induces differentiation of human embryonic stem cells to extraembryonic lineages. In: Stem cells (Dayton, Ohio), Jg. 23, H. 8, S. 1035–1043.

Ikenaka, Yasuhide; Yoshiji, Hitoshi; Kuriyama, Shigeki; Yoshii, Junichi; Noguchi, Ryuichi; Tsujinoue, Hirohisa et al. (2003): Tissue inhibitor of metalloproteinases-1 (TIMP-1) inhibits tumor growth and angiogenesis in the TIMP-1 transgenic mouse model. In: International journal of cancer. Journal international du cancer, Jg. 105, H. 3, S. 340–346.

Kaczmarek, E.; Koziak, K.; Sévigny, J.; Siegel, J. B.; Anrather, J.; Beaudoin, A. R. et al. (1996): Identification and characterization of CD39/vascular ATP diphosphohydrolase. In: The Journal of biological chemistry, Jg. 271, H. 51, S. 33116–33122.

Kadri, T.; Lataillade, J-J; Doucet, C.; Marie, A.; Ernou, I.; Bourin, P. et al. (2005): Proteomic study of Galectin-1 expression in human mesenchymal stem cells. In: Stem cells and development, Jg. 14, H. 2, S. 204–212.

Kessel, M.; Gruss, P. (1990): Murine developmental control genes. In: Science (New York, N.Y.), Jg. 249, H. 4967, S. 374–379.

Kessel, M.; Gruss, P. (1991): Homeotic transformations of murine vertebrae and concomitant alteration of Hox codes induced by retinoic acid. In: Cell, Jg. 67, H. 1, S. 89–104.

Kim, S. W.; Lajara, R.; Rotwein, P. (1991): Structure and function of a human insulin-like growth factor-I gene promoter. In: Molecular endocrinology (Baltimore, Md.), Jg. 5, H. 12, S. 1964–1972.

Kirchmair, R.; Hogue-Angeletti, R.; Gutierrez, J.; Fischer-Colbrie, R.; Winkler, H. (1993): Secretoneurin--a neuropeptide generated in brain, adrenal medulla and other endocrine tissues by proteolytic processing of secretogranin II (chromogranin C). In: Neuroscience, Jg. 53, H. 2, S. 359–365.

Klein, Walter M.; Wu, Bryan P.; Zhao, Shuping; Wu, Hong; Klein-Szanto, Andres J. P.; Tahan, Steven R. (2007): Increased expression of stem cell markers in malignant melanoma. In: Modern pathology : an official journal of the United States and Canadian Academy of Pathology, Inc, Jg. 20, H. 1, S. 102–107.

La Porta, Caterina A. M.; Porro, D.; Comolli, R. (2002): Higher levels of melanin and inhibition of cdk2 activity in primary human melanoma cells WM115 overexpressing nPKCdelta. In: Melanoma research, Jg. 12, H. 4, S. 297–307.

Laizé, Vincent; Martel, Paulo; Viegas, Carla S. B.; Price, Paul A.; Cancela, M. Leonor (2005): Evolution of matrix and bone gamma-carboxyglutamic acid proteins in vertebrates. In: The Journal of biological chemistry, Jg. 280, H. 29, S. 26659–26668.

Lee, Jonathan M. (2003): The role of protein elongation factor eEF1A2 in ovarian cancer. In: Reproductive biology and endocrinology : RB&E, Jg. 1, S. 69.

Lewis, E. B. (1978): A gene complex controlling segmentation in Drosophila. In: Nature, Jg. 276, H. 5688, S. 565–570.

Li, Li; Cicek, Mine S.; Casey, Graham; Witte, John S. (2004): No association between genetic polymorphisms in IGF-I and IGFBP-3 and prostate cancer. In: Cancer epidemiology, biomarkers & prevention : a publication of the American Association for Cancer Research, cosponsored by the American Society of Preventive Oncology, Jg. 13, H. 3, S. 497–498.

Li, R.; Wang, H.; Bekele, B. N.; Yin, Z.; Caraway, N. P.; Katz, R. L. et al. (2006): Identification of putative oncogenes in lung adenocarcinoma by a comprehensive functional genomic approach. In: Oncogene, Jg. 25, H. 18, S. 2628–2635.

Lin, Tongxiang; Chao, Connie; Saito, Shin'ichi; Mazur, Sharlyn J.; Murphy, Maureen E.; Appella, Ettore; Xu, Yang (2005): p53 induces differentiation of mouse embryonic stem cells by suppressing Nanog expression. In: Nature cell biology, Jg. 7, H. 2, S. 165–171.

Liu, Mingguang; Dai, Bingbing; Kang, Shin-Hyuk; Ban, Kechen; Huang, Feng-Ju; Lang, Frederick F. et al. (2006a): FoxM1B is overexpressed in human glioblastomas and critically regulates the tumorigenicity of glioma cells. In: Cancer research, Jg. 66, H. 7, S. 3593–3602.

Liu, Xu-Wen; Bernardo, M. Margarida; Fridman, Rafael; Kim, Hyeong-Reh Choi (2003): Tissue inhibitor of metalloproteinase-1 protects human breast epithelial cells against intrinsic apoptotic cell death via the focal adhesion kinase/phosphatidylinositol 3-kinase and MAPK signaling pathway. In: The Journal of biological chemistry, Jg. 278, H. 41, S. 40364–40372.

Liu, Y.; Borchert, G. L.; Surazynski, A.; Hu, C-A; Phang, J. M. (2006b): Proline oxidase activates both intrinsic and extrinsic pathways for apoptosis: the role of ROS/superoxides, NFAT and MEK/ERK signaling. In: Oncogene, Jg. 25, H. 41, S. 5640–5647.

Loh, Yuin-Han; Ng, Jia-Hui; Ng, Huck-Hui (2008): Molecular framework underlying pluripotency. In: Cell cycle (Georgetown, Tex.), Jg. 7, H. 7, S. 885–891.

Looijenga, Leendert H. J.; Stoop, Hans; Leeuw, Hubert P. J. C. de; Gouveia Brazao, Carlos A. de; Gillis, Ad J. M.; van Roozendaal, Kees E. P. et al. (2003): POU5F1 (OCT3/4) identifies cells with pluripotent potential in human germ cell tumors. In: Cancer research, Jg. 63, H. 9, S. 2244–2250.

Lund, A.; Knudsen, S. M.; Vissing, H.; Clark, B.; Tommerup, N. (1996): Assignment of human elongation factor 1alpha genes: EEF1A maps to chromosome 6q14 and EEF1A2 to 20q13.3. In: Genomics, Jg. 36, H. 2, S. 359–361.

Maeda, Kazuhiko; Hamada, Jun-Ichi; Takahashi, Yoko; Tada, Mitsuhiro; Yamamoto, Yuhei; Sugihara, Tsuneki; Moriuchi, Tetsuya (2005): Altered expressions of HOX genes in human cutaneous malignant melanoma. In: International journal of cancer. Journal international du cancer, Jg. 114, H. 3, S. 436–441.

Maliszewski, C. R.; Delespesse, G. J.; Schoenborn, M. A.; Armitage, R. J.; Fanslow, W. C.; Nakajima, T. et al. (1994): The CD39 lymphoid cell activation antigen. Molecular cloning and structural characterization. In: Journal of immunology (Baltimore, Md. : 1950), Jg. 153, H. 8, S. 3574–3583.

Martin, I.; Jakob, M.; Schäfer, D.; Dick, W.; Spagnoli, G.; Heberer, M. (2001): Quantitative analysis of gene expression in human articular cartilage from normal and osteoarthritic joints. In: Osteoarthritis and cartilage / OARS, Osteoarthritis Research Society, Jg. 9, H. 2, S. 112–118.

Maxwell, Steve A.; Rivera, Armando (2003): Proline oxidase induces apoptosis in tumor cells, and its expression is frequently absent or reduced in renal carcinomas. In: The Journal of biological chemistry, Jg. 278, H. 11, S. 9784–9789.

McGinnis, W.; Krumlauf, R. (1992): Homeobox genes and axial patterning. In: Cell, Jg. 68, H. 2, S. 283–302.

McIntyre, Daniel C.; Rakshit, Sabita; Yallowitz, Alisha R.; Loken, Luke; Jeannotte, Lucie; Capecchi, Mario R.; Wellik, Deneen M. (2007): Hox patterning of the vertebrate rib cage. In: Development (Cambridge, England), Jg. 134, H. 16, S. 2981–2989.

Missmer, Stacey A.; Haiman, Christopher A.; Hunter, David J.; Willett, Walter C.; Colditz, Graham A.; Speizer, Frank E. et al. (2002): A sequence repeat in the insulin-like growth factor-1 gene and risk of breast cancer. In: International journal of cancer. Journal international du cancer, Jg. 100, H. 3, S. 332–336.

Mizumoto, Norikatsu; Kumamoto, Tadashi; Robson, Simon C.; Sévigny, Jean; Matsue, Hiroyuki; Enjyoji, Keiichi; Takashima, Akira (2002): CD39 is the dominant Langerhans cell-associated ecto-NTPDase: modulatory roles in inflammation and immune responsiveness. In: Nature medicine, Jg. 8, H. 4, S. 358–365.

Monzani, Elena; Facchetti, Floriana; Galmozzi, Enrico; Corsini, Elena; Benetti, Anna; Cavazzin, Chiara et al. (2007): Melanoma contains CD133 and ABCG2 positive cells with enhanced tumourigenic potential. In: European journal of cancer (Oxford, England : 1990), Jg. 43, H. 5, S. 935–946.

Morgan, Richard; Pirard, Patricia Macanas; Shears, Liesl; Sohal, Jastinder; Pettengell, Ruth; Pandha, Hardev S. (2007): Antagonism of HOX/PBX dimer formation blocks the in vivo proliferation of melanoma. In: Cancer research, Jg. 67, H. 12, S. 5806–5813.

Morimoto, Libby M.; Newcomb, Polly A.; White, Emily; Bigler, Jeannette; Potter, John D. (2005): Insulin-like growth factor polymorphisms and colorectal cancer risk. In: Cancer epidemiology, biomarkers & prevention : a publication of the American Association for Cancer Research, cosponsored by the American Society of Preventive Oncology, Jg. 14, H. 5, S. 1204–1211.

Murdoch, Barbara; Chadwick, Kristin; Martin, Matthew; Shojaei, Farbod; Shah, Kavita V.; Gallacher, Lisa et al. (2003): Wnt-5A augments repopulating capacity and primitive hematopoietic development of human blood stem cells in vivo. In: Proceedings of the National Academy of Sciences of the United States of America, Jg. 100, H. 6, S. 3422–3427.

Nam, Robert K.; Trachtenberg, John; Jewett, Michael A. S.; Toi, Ants; Evans, Andrew; Emami, Marjan et al. (2005): Serum insulin-like growth factor-I levels and prostatic intraepithelial neoplasia: a clue to the relationship between IGF-I physiology and prostate cancer risk. In: Cancer epidemiology, biomarkers & prevention : a publication of the American Association for Cancer Research, cosponsored by the American Society of Preventive Oncology, Jg. 14, H. 5, S. 1270–1273.

Neumaier, M.; Paululat, S.; Chan, A.; Matthaes, P.; Wagener, C. (1993): Biliary glycoprotein, a potential human cell adhesion molecule, is down-regulated in colorectal carcinomas. In: Proceedings of the National Academy of Sciences of the United States of America, Jg. 90, H. 22, S. 10744–10748.

Neuzil, Jiri; Stantic, Marina; Zobalova, Renata; Chladova, Jaromira; Wang, Xiufang; Prochazka, Lubomir et al. (2007): Tumour-initiating cells vs. cancer 'stem' cells and CD133: what's in the name? In: Biochemical and biophysical research communications, Jg. 355, H. 4, S. 855–859.

O'Brien, Catherine A.; Pollett, Aaron; Gallinger, Steven; Dick, John E. (2007): A human colon cancer cell capable of initiating tumour growth in immunodeficient mice. In: Nature, Jg. 445, H. 7123, S. 106–110.

Orend, G.; Chiquet-Ehrismann, R. (2000): Adhesion modulation by antiadhesive molecules of the extracellular matrix. In: Experimental cell research, Jg. 261, H. 1, S. 104–110.

Otsubo, T.; Akiyama, Y.; Yanagihara, K.; Yuasa, Y. (2008): SOX2 is frequently downregulated in gastric cancers and inhibits cell growth through cell-cycle arrest and apoptosis. In: British journal of cancer, Jg. 98, H. 4, S. 824–831.

Pace, K. E.; Hahn, H. P.; Pang, M.; Nguyen, J. T.; Baum, L. G. (2000): CD7 delivers a pro-apoptotic signal during galectin-1-induced T cell death. In: Journal of immunology (Baltimore, Md. : 1950), Jg. 165, H. 5, S. 2331–2334.

Pace, K. E.; Lee, C.; Stewart, P. L.; Baum, L. G. (1999): Restricted receptor segregation into membrane microdomains occurs on human T cells during apoptosis induced by galectin-1. In: Journal of immunology (Baltimore, Md. : 1950), Jg. 163, H. 7, S. 3801–3811.

Pan, Guangjin; Thomson, James A. (2007): Nanog and transcriptional networks in embryonic stem cell pluripotency. In: Cell research, Jg. 17, H. 1, S. 42–49.

Pandhare, Jui; Cooper, Sandra K.; Phang, James M. (2006): Proline oxidase, a proapoptotic gene, is induced by troglitazone: evidence for both peroxisome proliferator-activated receptor gamma-dependent and -independent mechanisms. In: The Journal of biological chemistry, Jg. 281, H. 4, S. 2044–2052.

Pardal, Ricardo; Clarke, Michael F.; Morrison, Sean J. (2003): Applying the principles of stem-cell biology to cancer. In: Nature reviews. Cancer, Jg. 3, H. 12, S. 895–902.

Perillo, N. L.; Marcus, M. E.; Baum, L. G. (1998): Galectins: versatile modulators of cell adhesion, cell proliferation, and cell death. In: Journal of molecular medicine (Berlin, Germany), Jg. 76, H. 6, S. 402–412.

Perillo, N. L.; Pace, K. E.; Seilhamer, J. J.; Baum, L. G. (1995): Apoptosis of T cells mediated by galectin-1. In: Nature, Jg. 378, H. 6558, S. 736–739.

Pfaffl, M. W. (2001): A new mathematical model for relative quantification in real-time RT-PCR. In: Nucleic acids research, Jg. 29, H. 9, S. e45.

Playford, M. P.; Bicknell, D.; Bodmer, W. F.; Macaulay, V. M. (2000): Insulin-like growth factor 1 regulates the location, stability, and transcriptional activity of beta-catenin. In: Proceedings of the National Academy of Sciences of the United States of America, Jg. 97, H. 22, S. 12103–12108.

Pouysségur, Jacques; Dayan, Frédéric; Mazure, Nathalie M. (2006): Hypoxia signalling in cancer and approaches to enforce tumour regression. In: Nature, Jg. 441, H. 7092, S. 437–443.

Prenzel, Klaus L.; Warnecke-Eberz, Ute; Xi, Huan; Brabender, Jan; Baldus, Stephan E.; Bollschweiler, Elfriede et al. (2006): Significant overexpression of SPARC/osteonectin mRNA in pancreatic cancer compared to cancer of the papilla of Vater. In: Oncology reports, Jg. 15, H. 5, S. 1397–1401.

Price, P. A.; Rice, J. S.; Williamson, M. K. (1994): Conserved phosphorylation of serines in the Ser-X-Glu/Ser(P) sequences of the vitamin K-dependent matrix Gla protein from shark, lamb, rat, cow, and human. In: Protein science : a publication of the Protein Society, Jg. 3, H. 5, S. 822–830.

Qiang, Ya-Wei; Endo, Yoshimi; Rubin, Jeffrey S.; Rudikoff, Stuart (2003): Wnt signaling in B-cell neoplasia. In: Oncogene, Jg. 22, H. 10, S. 1536–1545.

Reya, T.; Morrison, S. J.; Clarke, M. F.; Weissman, I. L. (2001): Stem cells, cancer, and cancer stem cells. In: Nature, Jg. 414, H. 6859, S. 105–111.

Ricci-Vitiani, Lucia; Lombardi, Dario G.; Pilozzi, Emanuela; Biffoni, Mauro; Todaro, Matilde; Peschle, Cesare; Maria, Ruggero de (2007): Identification and expansion of human colon-cancer-initiating cells. In: Nature, Jg. 445, H. 7123, S. 111–115.

Richardson, Gavin D.; Robson, Craig N.; Lang, Shona H.; Neal, David E.; Maitland, Norman J.; Collins, Anne T. (2004): CD133, a novel marker for human prostatic epithelial stem cells. In: Journal of cell science, Jg. 117, H. Pt 16, S. 3539–3545.

Rietschel, Petra; Wolchok, Jedd D.; Krown, Susan; Gerst, Scott; Jungbluth, Achim A.; Busam, Klaus et al. (2008): Phase II study of extended-dose temozolomide in patients with melanoma. In: Journal of clinical oncology : official journal of the American Society of Clinical Oncology, Jg. 26, H. 14, S. 2299–2304.

Ruangpratheep, Chetana; Lohachittranond, Chanida; Poonpracha, Tara; Punyarit, Phaibul (2005): OCT4 expression on a case of poorly differentiated (insular) carcinoma of the thyroid gland and minireview. In: Journal of the Medical Association of Thailand = Chotmaihet thangphaet, Jg. 88 Suppl 3, S. S281-9.

Rubin, M. R.; King, W.; Toth, L. E.; Sawczuk, I. S.; Levine, M. S.; D'Eustachio, P.; Nguyen-Huu, M. C. (1987): Murine Hox-1.7 homeo-box gene: cloning, chromosomal location, and expression. In: Molecular and cellular biology, Jg. 7, H. 10, S. 3836–3841.

Ruiz, Christian; Huang, Wentao; Hegi, Monika E.; Lange, Katrin; Hamou, Marie-France; Fluri, Erika et al. (2004): Growth promoting signaling by tenascin-C [corrected]. In: Cancer research, Jg. 64, H. 20, S. 7377–7385.

Sabatino, Marianna; Stroncek, David F.; Klein, Harvey; Marincola, Francesco M.; Wang, Ena (2009): Stem cells in melanoma development. In: Cancer letters, Jg. 279, H. 2, S. 119–125.

Sadej, Rafal; Inai, Kunihiro; Rajfur, Zenon; Ostapkowicz, Anna; Kohler, Jon; Skladanowski, Andrzej C. et al. (2008): Tenascin C interacts with ecto-5'-nucleotidase (eN) and regulates adenosine generation in cancer cells. In: Biochimica et biophysica acta, Jg. 1782, H. 1, S. 35–40.

Sakaguchi, Masanori; Shingo, Tetsuro; Shimazaki, Takuya; Okano, Hirotaka James; Shiwa, Mieko; Ishibashi, Satoru et al. (2006): A carbohydrate-binding protein, Galectin-1, promotes proliferation of adult neural stem cells. In: Proceedings of the National Academy of Sciences of the United States of America, Jg. 103, H. 18, S. 7112–7117.

Salmaggi, Andrea; Boiardi, Amerigo; Gelati, Maurizio; Russo, Annamaria; Calatozzolo, Chiara; Ciusani, Emilio et al. (2006): Glioblastoma-derived tumorospheres identify a population of tumor stem-like cells with angiogenic potential and enhanced multidrug resistance phenotype. In: Glia, Jg. 54, H. 8, S. 850–860.

Santonocito, Concetta; Paradisi, Andrea; Capizzi, Rodolfo; Concolino, Paola; Lavieri, Maria Michela; Lanza Silveri, Sara et al. (2008): Insulin-like growth factor I (CA) repeats are associated with higher melanoma's Breslow index but not associated with the presence of the melanoma. A pilot study. In: Clinica chimica acta; international journal of clinical chemistry, Jg. 390, H. 1-2, S. 104–109.

Schaffer, Andrea; Koushik, Anita; Trottier, Helen; Duarte-Franco, Eliane; Mansour, Nabil; Arseneau, Jocelyne et al. (2007): Insulin-like growth factor-I and risk of high-grade cervical intraepithelial neoplasia. In: Cancer epidemiology, biomarkers & prevention : a publication of the American Association for Cancer Research, cosponsored by the American Society of Preventive Oncology, Jg. 16, H. 4, S. 716–722.

Schatton, Tobias; Murphy, George F.; Frank, Natasha Y.; Yamaura, Kazuhiro; Waaga-Gasser, Ana Maria; Gasser, Martin et al. (2008): Identification of cells initiating human melanomas. In: Nature, Jg. 451, H. 7176, S. 345–349.

Schildkraut, Joellen M.; Demark-Wahnefried, Wendy; Wenham, Robert M.; Grubber, Janet; Jeffreys, Amy S.; Grambow, Steven C. et al. (2005): IGF1 (CA)19 repeat and IGFBP3 -202 A/C genotypes and the risk of prostate cancer in Black and White men. In: Cancer epidemiology, biomarkers & prevention : a publication of the American Association for Cancer Research, cosponsored by the American Society of Preventive Oncology, Jg. 14, H. 2, S. 403–408.

Schlenska-Lange, Anke; Knüpfer, Heike; Lange, Tobias J.; Kiess, Wieland; Knüpfer, Matthias: Cell proliferation and migration in glioblastoma multiforme cell lines are influenced by insulin-like growth factor I in vitro. In: Anticancer research, Jg. 28, H. 2A, S. 1055–1060.

Schneider, Adele; Bardakjian, Tanya M.; Zhou, Jie; Hughes, Nkecha; Keep, Rosanne; Dorsainville, Darnelle et al. (2008): Familial recurrence of SOX2 anophthalmia syndrome: phenotypically normal mother with two affected daughters. In: American journal of medical genetics. Part A, Jg. 146A, H. 21, S. 2794–2798.

Schurgers, L. J.; Spronk, H. M. H.; Skepper, J. N.; Hackeng, T. M.; Shanahan, C. M.; Vermeer, C. et al. (2007): Post-translational modifications regulate matrix Gla protein function: importance for inhibition of vascular smooth muscle cell calcification. In: Journal of thrombosis and haemostasis : JTH, Jg. 5, H. 12, S. 2503–2511.

Sell, S. (1993): Cellular origin of cancer: dedifferentiation or stem cell maturation arrest? In: Environmental health perspectives, Jg. 101 Suppl 5, S. 15–26.

Sell, S.; Pierce, G. B. (1994): Maturation arrest of stem cell differentiation is a common pathway for the cellular origin of teratocarcinomas and epithelial cancers. In: Laboratory investigation; a journal of technical methods and pathology, Jg. 70, H. 1, S. 6–22.

Sell, Stewart (2004): Stem cell origin of cancer and differentiation therapy. In: Critical reviews in oncology/hematology, Jg. 51, H. 1, S. 1–28.

Sharma, Sameer; Tammela, Jonathan; Wang, Xinhui; Arnouk, Hilal; Driscoll, Deborah; Mhawech-Fauceglia, Paulette et al. (2007): Characterization of a putative ovarian oncogene, elongation factor 1alpha, isolated by panning a synthetic phage display single-chain variable fragment library with cultured human ovarian cancer cells. In: Clinical cancer research : an official journal of the American Association for Cancer Research, Jg. 13, H. 19, S. 5889–5896.

Sharrock, C. E.; Kaminski, E.; Man, S. (1990): Limiting dilution analysis of human T cells: a useful clinical tool. In: Immunology today, Jg. 11, H. 8, S. 281–286.

Shi, Yanhong; Sun, Guoqiang; Zhao, Chunnian; Stewart, Richard (2008): Neural stem cell self-renewal. In: Critical reviews in oncology/hematology, Jg. 65, H. 1, S. 43–53.

Shyu, Woei-Cherng; Lin, Shinn-Zong; Chiang, Ming-Fu; Chen, Der-Cherng; Su, Ching-Yuan; Wang, Hsiao-Jung et al. (2008): Secretoneurin promotes neuroprotection and neuronal plasticity via the Jak2/Stat3 pathway in murine models of stroke. In: The Journal of clinical investigation, Jg. 118, H. 1, S. 133–148.

Singh, Sheila; Dirks, Peter B. (2007): Brain tumor stem cells: identification and concepts. In: Neurosurgery clinics of North America, Jg. 18, H. 1, S. 31-8, viii.

Singh, Sheila K.; Clarke, Ian D.; Hide, Takuichiro; Dirks, Peter B. (2004a): Cancer stem cells in nervous system tumors. In: Oncogene, Jg. 23, H. 43, S. 7267–7273.

Singh, Sheila K.; Clarke, Ian D.; Terasaki, Mizuhiko; Bonn, Victoria E.; Hawkins, Cynthia; Squire, Jeremy; Dirks, Peter B. (2003): Identification of a cancer stem cell in human brain tumors. In: Cancer research, Jg. 63, H. 18, S. 5821–5828.

Singh, Sheila K.; Hawkins, Cynthia; Clarke, Ian D.; Squire, Jeremy A.; Bayani, Jane; Hide, Takuichiro et al. (2004b): Identification of human brain tumour initiating cells. In: Nature, Jg. 432, H. 7015, S. 396–401.

Situm, Mirna; Buljan, Marija; Bulić, Suzana Otanić; Simić, Dubravka (2007): The mechanisms of UV radiation in the development of malignant melanoma. In: Collegium antropologicum, Jg. 31 Suppl 1, S. 13–16.

Slattery, Martha L.; Samowitz, Wade; Curtin, Karen; Ma, Khe Ni; Hoffman, Michael; Caan, Bette; Neuhausen, Susan (2004): Associations among IRS1, IRS2, IGF1, and IGFBP3 genetic polymorphisms and colorectal cancer. In: Cancer epidemiology, biomarkers & prevention : a publication of the American Association for Cancer Research, cosponsored by the American Society of Preventive Oncology, Jg. 13, H. 7, S. 1206–1214.

Spagnoli, G. C.; Schaefer, C.; Willimann, T. E.; Kocher, T.; Amoroso, A.; Juretic, A. et al. (1995): Peptide-specific CTL in tumor infiltrating lymphocytes from metastatic melanomas expressing MART-1/Melan-A, gp100 and Tyrosinase genes: a study in an unselected group of HLA-A2.1-positive patients. In: International journal of cancer. Journal international du cancer, Jg. 64, H. 5, S. 309–315.

Spring, J.; Beck, K.; Chiquet-Ehrismann, R. (1989): Two contrary functions of tenascin: dissection of the active sites by recombinant tenascin fragments. In: Cell, Jg. 59, H. 2, S. 325–334.

Sun, Yu; Li, Huai; Yang, Henry; Rao, Mahendra S.; Zhan, Ming (2006): Mechanisms controlling embryonic stem cell self-renewal and differentiation. In: Critical reviews in eukaryotic gene expression, Jg. 16, H. 3, S. 211–231.

Suzuki, H.; Kawai, J.; Taga, C.; Yaoi, T.; Hara, A.; Hirose, K. et al. (1996): Stac, a novel neuron-specific protein with cysteine-rich and SH3 domains. In: Biochemical and biophysical research communications, Jg. 229, H. 3, S. 902–909.

Svedmyr, E.; Ernberg, I.; Seeley, J.; Weiland, O.; Masucci, G.; Tsukuda, K. et al. (1984): Virologic, immunologic, and clinical observations on a patient during the incubation, acute, and convalescent phases of infectious mononucleosis. In: Clinical immunology and immunopathology, Jg. 30, H. 3, S. 437–450.

Svingen, Terje; Tonissen, Kathryn F.: Altered HOX gene expression in human skin and breast cancer cells. In: Cancer biology & therapy, Jg. 2, H. 5, S. 518–523.

Taipale, J.; Beachy, P. A. (2001): The Hedgehog and Wnt signalling pathways in cancer. In: Nature, Jg. 411, H. 6835, S. 349–354.

Taswell, C. (1981): Limiting dilution assays for the determination of immunocompetent cell frequencies. I. Data analysis. In: Journal of immunology (Baltimore, Md. : 1950), Jg. 126, H. 4, S. 1614–1619.

Tavaluc, Raluca T.; Hart, Lori S.; Dicker, David T.; El-Deiry, Wafik S. (2007): Effects of low confluency, serum starvation and hypoxia on the side population of cancer cell lines. In: Cell cycle (Georgetown, Tex.), Jg. 6, H. 20, S. 2554–2562.

Tsuchiya, Norihiko; Wang, Lizhong; Horikawa, Yohei; Inoue, Takamitsu; Kakinuma, Hideaki; Matsuura, Shinobu et al. (2005): CA repeat polymorphism in the insulin-like growth factor-I gene is associated with increased risk of prostate cancer and benign prostatic hyperplasia. In: International journal of oncology, Jg. 26, H. 1, S. 225–231.

van de Wetering, Marc; Sancho, Elena; Verweij, Cornelis; Lau, Wim de; Oving, Irma; Hurlstone, Adam et al. (2002): The beta-catenin/TCF-4 complex imposes a crypt progenitor phenotype on colorectal cancer cells. In: Cell, Jg. 111, H. 2, S. 241–250.

van den Brûle, F. A.; Buicu, C.; Baldet, M.; Sobel, M. E.; Cooper, D. N.; Marschal, P.; Castronovo, V. (1995): Galectin-1 modulates human melanoma cell adhesion to laminin. In: Biochemical and biophysical research communications, Jg. 209, H. 2, S. 760–767.

Vaughan, Hilary A.; Svobodova, Suzanne; Macgregor, Duncan; Sturrock, Sue; Jungbluth, Achim A.; Browning, Judy et al. (2004): Immunohistochemical and molecular analysis of human melanomas for expression of the human cancer-testis antigens NY-ESO-1 and LAGE-

1. In: Clinical cancer research : an official journal of the American Association for Cancer Research, Jg. 10, H. 24, S. 8396–8404.

Vita, G. de; Barba, P.; Odartchenko, N.; Givel, J. C.; Freschi, G.; Bucciarelli, G. et al. (1993): Expression of homeobox-containing genes in primary and metastatic colorectal cancer. In: European journal of cancer (Oxford, England : 1990), Jg. 29A, H. 6, S. 887–893.

Wagner, Kerstin; Hemminki, Kari; Grzybowska, Ewa; Klaes, Rüdiger; Butkiewicz, Dorota; Pamula, Jolanta et al. (2004): The insulin-like growth factor-1 pathway mediator genes: SHC1 Met300Val shows a protective effect in breast cancer. In: Carcinogenesis, Jg. 25, H. 12, S. 2473–2478.

Walzel, H.; Schulz, U.; Neels, P.; Brock, J. (1999): Galectin-1, a natural ligand for the receptor-type protein tyrosine phosphatase CD45. In: Immunology letters, Jg. 67, H. 3, S. 193–202.

Ward, Ryan J.; Dirks, Peter B. (2007): Cancer stem cells: at the headwaters of tumor development. In: Annual review of pathology, Jg. 2, S. 175–189.

Wechsler-Reya, R.; Scott, M. P. (2001): The developmental biology of brain tumors. In: Annual review of neuroscience, Jg. 24, S. 385–428.

Wechsler-Reya, R. J. (2001): Caught in the matrix: how vitronectin controls neuronal differentiation. In: Trends in neurosciences, Jg. 24, H. 12, S. 680–682.

Wen, Wanqing; Gao, Yu-Tang; Shu, Xiao-Ou; Yu, Herbert; Cai, Qiuyin; Smith, Jeffrey R.; Zheng, Wei (2005): Insulin-like growth factor-I gene polymorphism and breast cancer risk in Chinese women. In: International journal of cancer. Journal international du cancer, Jg. 113, H. 2, S. 307–311.

Willert, Karl; Brown, Jeffrey D.; Danenberg, Esther; Duncan, Andrew W.; Weissman, Irving L.; Reya, Tannishtha et al. (2003): Wnt proteins are lipid-modified and can act as stem cell growth factors. In: Nature, Jg. 423, H. 6938, S. 448–452.

Wong, Hui-Lee; Delellis, Katherine; Probst-Hensch, Nicole; Koh, Woon-Puay; van Den Berg, David; Lee, Hin-Peng et al. (2005): A new single nucleotide polymorphism in the insulin-like growth factor I regulatory region associates with colorectal cancer risk in singapore chinese. In: Cancer epidemiology, biomarkers & prevention : a publication of the American Association for Cancer Research, cosponsored by the American Society of Preventive Oncology, Jg. 14, H. 1, S. 144–151.

Yao, Yucheng; Shahbazian, Ani; Boström, Kristina I. (2008a): Proline and gamma-carboxylated glutamate residues in matrix Gla protein are critical for binding of bone morphogenetic protein-4. In: Circulation research, Jg. 102, H. 9, S. 1065–1074.

Yao, Yucheng; Shao, Esther S.; Jumabay, Medet; Shahbazian, Ani; Ji, Sheng; Boström, Kristina I. (2008b): High-density lipoproteins affect endothelial BMP-signaling by modulating expression of the activin-like kinase receptor 1 and 2. In: Arteriosclerosis, thrombosis, and vascular biology, Jg. 28, H. 12, S. 2266–2274.

Yasuda, Shin-ya; Tsuneyoshi, Norihiro; Sumi, Tomoyuki; Hasegawa, Kouichi; Tada, Takashi; Nakatsuji, Norio; Suemori, Hirofumi (2006): NANOG maintains self-renewal of primate ES cells in the absence of a feeder layer. In: Genes to cells : devoted to molecular & cellular mechanisms, Jg. 11, H. 9, S. 1115–1123.

Yu, H.; Berkel, H. (1999): Insulin-like growth factors and cancer. In: The Journal of the Louisiana State Medical Society : official organ of the Louisiana State Medical Society, Jg. 151, H. 4, S. 218–223.

Yu, H.; Rohan, T. (2000): Role of the insulin-like growth factor family in cancer development and progression. In: Journal of the National Cancer Institute, Jg. 92, H. 18, S. 1472–1489.

Zhou, Jiangbing; Zhang, Ying (2008): Cancer stem cells: Models, mechanisms and implications for improved treatment. In: Cell cycle (Georgetown, Tex.), Jg. 7, H. 10, S. 1360–1370.

Zhu, Fan; Li, Wen-Xin; Jiang, Da-He; Gou, De-Ming (2002): Differential expression of the Quox-1 gene in normal human cells, early human embryo, and tumor cells. In: Cell and tissue research, Jg. 308, H. 2, S. 333–337.

Zhu, Yuan; Parada, Luis F. (2002): The molecular and genetic basis of neurological tumours. In: Nature reviews. Cancer, Jg. 2, H. 8, S. 616–626.

Zurawel, R. H.; Chiappa, S. A.; Allen, C.; Raffel, C. (1998): Sporadic medulloblastomas contain oncogenic beta-catenin mutations. In: Cancer research, Jg. 58, H. 5, S. 896–899.

APPENDIX

ACKNOWLEDGEMENTS

It's a pleasure to thank those who made this thesis possible.

Most importantly, this dissertation and the associated stay abroad in Switzerland would not have been possible without the support and patience of my family to whom this dissertation is dedicated to. They all have been a constant source of motivation and strength all these years. I would like to express my gratitude especially to my parents **Dr. Hans-Peter** and **Carolina Pia Zimmerer**.

I owe my deepest gratitude to my advisor **Prof. Dr. Giulio C. Spagnoli**, the head of the **Oncology Surgery** group of the Institute for Surgical Research (ICFS) at the University Hospital Basel in Switzerland for his guidance, patience and support over three years. His wisdom, knowledge and commitment to the highest standards inspired and motivated me. Thank you, Giulio, for your consistent notations in my writings and for carefully reading and commenting on countless revisions of this manuscript.

I am heartly thankful to my co-advisor **Dr. Andrea Barbero** from the **Tissue Engineering** group whose encouragement, supervision and support from the preliminary to the concluding level enabled me to develop an understanding of the subject. I am deeply grateful to him for the long discussions that helped me sort out the technical details of my work. Mille gracie!

I am also indebted to all members of the **Oncology Surgery** group and to **Prof. Dr. Ivan Martin`s Tissue Engineering** group with whom I have interacted during my time in the Lab. Thank you all for your support, insightful comments and constructive criticisms at different stages of my research!

I am grateful to **Prof. Dr. Clemente Cillo** und **Dr Giulia Schiavo** from the Pathology at the University Hospital Basel who provided assistance in analysing the HOX gene expression. I also would like to sincerely thank **Dr. Philippe Demougin** from the **Biozentrum** Basel for his guidance on the acquisition of the micro array data.

I would also like to give a special reference to **Prof. Dr. Dr. Ralf Schön** from the Department of Cranio-maxillofacial Surgery at the University Hospital Freiburg who agreed to supervise the thesis at my faculty and to write the primary expert opinion on my dissertation.

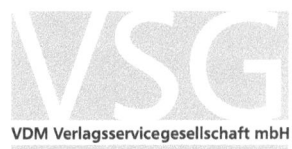

Die VDM Verlagsservicegesellschaft sucht für wissenschaftliche Verlage abgeschlossene und herausragende

Dissertationen, Habilitationen, Diplomarbeiten, Master Theses, Magisterarbeiten usw.

für die kostenlose Publikation als Fachbuch.

Sie verfügen über eine Arbeit, die hohen inhaltlichen und formalen Ansprüchen genügt, und haben Interesse an einer honorarvergüteten Publikation?

Dann senden Sie bitte erste Informationen über sich und Ihre Arbeit per Email an *info@vdm-vsg.de*.

Sie erhalten kurzfristig unser Feedback!

VDM Verlagsservicegesellschaft mbH
Dudweiler Landstr. 99
D - 66123 Saarbrücken

Telefon +49 681 3720 174
Fax +49 681 3720 1749

www.vdm-vsg.de

Die VDM Verlagsservicegesellschaft mbH vertritt

 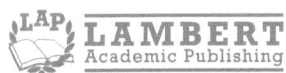 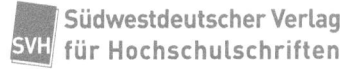

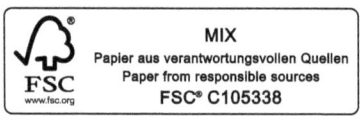

Printed by Books on Demand GmbH, Norderstedt / Germany